THE DAY
THE
SCIENCE
DIED

COVID VACCINES AND THE POWER OF FEAR

Expert Endorsements

"A gut-wrenching account of the harms caused by COVID-19 vaccines in diverse populations of healthy people who willingly took these experimental and half-baked jabs. A meticulous documentation of what is wrong with agencies that are supposed to safeguard our health interests and how the system is set up so that it can be easily gamed. Morality and ethics are in name only. The book outlines so many reasons as to why we need a 'reset' for biomedical science and the practice of medicine. A must read."

ADITI BHARGAVA, *Ph.D., Prof. Emeritus, UCSF*

"No one ever thinks something will happen to them until it does. Harms in medicine often go invisible. I learned long ago the importance of sharing our stories. Not only is it healing, but lets others know they're not alone. Collectively, our stories speak truth to power and can drive change. Never let anyone take your story away from you."

KIM WITCZAK, *Global Drug Safety Advocate and FDA Consumer Representative*

"Kudos to Patrick Hahn for outlining the history of the Covid "vaccine" and how we have been herded like sheep to the slaughter over the past several years by huge, evil corporations. His conclusions echo my own in Cassandra's Memo: Covid and the Global Psychopaths (2022). Do not miss this well-written and exhaustively referenced work if you want to learn the truth."

ROBERT YOHO, *M.D., author of Butchered by Healthcare*

"In his thoroughly researched book, Patrick Hahn sets out the perils of the pandemic and our nation's disastrous policy response—the emergency authorization of the novel, inadequately tested mRNA vaccine. A mesmerizing time-capsule of the vaccine's mass roll-out, Hahn also reveals the hidden human collateral of the vaccine's rushed approval, including his own injuries. Hahn outs the truth in this extraordinary documentation of conflicted interests, censorship, and propaganda ruling the agencies and individuals intended to protect us."

LINDA WASTILA, *M.S.P.H., Ph.D, Professor and Endowed Chair, University of Maryland Baltimore*

Also by Patrick D. Hahn

Obedience Pills

ADHD and the Medicalization of Childhood

Prescription for Sorrow

Antidepressants, Suicide and Violence

Madness and Genetic Determinism

Is Mental Illness in Our Genes?

THE DAY
THE
SCIENCE
DIED

COVID VACCINES AND THE POWER OF FEAR

PATRICK D. HAHN

Samizdat Health

Samizdat Health Writer's Co-operative Inc.

Cover Design: Samizdat Health / Photo collage: iStock, LightFieldStudios, fergregory

First Printing, 2023

Title: The Day the Science Died

ISBN: 978-1-989963-30-2

Publisher: Samizdat Health Writer's Co-operative Inc.

www.samizdathealth.org

www.patrickhahn.net

For Ethan, Nana Konadu, and Katie

Contents

Prologue

27 November 2020

It was the day after Thanksgiving, an unseasonably warm afternoon, the rolling hills and dales of Washington County forming a viridescent backdrop to the last remaining golden leaves of autumn still clinging to the trees. It was a perfect day for the Old Man to go for a walk with his nephew and nieces, who in turn were the perfect ages for such an undertaking—old enough to be able to carry on an intelligent conversation, and yet young enough still actually to want to spend time with the Old Man.

The four of them had barely gotten underway when they spotted a couple, a man and a woman, a couple of hundred yards away. Then the middle child, a girl, spoke up.

"We need to go back," she informed the Old Man solemnly. "We'll get the corona."

It was at that moment that I knew I had to do something. But what? Where to start?

In my second career as a science writer, I had published books on the history of psychiatric genetics and on antidepressants and violence, and was beginning my third book, on the toxic effects of the drugs commonly prescribed for something called "ADHD"—but the current crisis has taken things to a whole new level.

The coronavirus pandemic—and our society's panicky, scared response to that pandemic—has hit the nation and the world like a tsunami, so much so that history seems to divide into pre- and post-covid. We have entered Bizarro World, in which all the things that allow us to co-exist as a civilization of intelligent, self-governing men and women—work, school, church, fresh air, outdoor exercise, entrepreneurship, love, friendship, verve, spontaneity, joyous celebration, the human face—have been relentlessly downgraded. In place we are offered shame, blame, snitching, tattling, and a fear that pervades every facet of our existence. The very lifeblood of modern medicine—early detection and treatment of illness—has been systematically discredited, in favor of experimental shots using a kind of technology never before deployed on a large scale, and hundreds of millions of people have been induced or coerced into having these products injected into their bodies without any good idea of the benefits and risks. Even the meanings of key terms—such as "quarantine," "herd immunity," "anti-vaxxer," and "vaccine" itself—have been altered, without any discussion or debate.

This is a crisis that touches upon every facet of our existence. Going from writing about antidepressants to writing about the covid is like going from swimming laps in a pool to being parachuted into the middle of the Pacific Ocean.

So when David Healy suggested in a telephone conversation that I write a book about the covid shots, I agreed immediately. This was a project I could sink my teeth into.

In order to keep this work of manageable length, I have confined my discussion to two products called "vaccines"—the only two such products generally available in the United States—and the attempts of the drugmakers and government agencies to exaggerate the benefits and hide the harms of these products. I also go into some detail about censorship and deplatforming of those who hold views dissenting from the official narrative concerning these matters, as well as government and media hate campaigns against "anti-vaxxers"—a term which now seemingly includes anyone who has any concerns about the safety and effectiveness of any product called a "vaccine" (and always remember, they had to change the definition of "vaccine" for these patented products to be called that). I do not examine the ethics of vaccine mandates in general.

For my part, I am a university teacher by profession. I have spent my entire career working to make scientific knowledge available to all. I have no formal training in medicine or public health. I have never claimed that my degree gives me any authority in these matters, but it has given me a perspective which, I believe, is undervalued.

I have long regarded with distaste the currently fashionable view of ourselves as fragile creatures who need huge amounts of expensive medical interventions from cradle to grave to keep us alive. My background is in evolutionary biology, and two things are perfectly obvious to me: 1) we evolved to thrive, and 2) we evolved to thrive *for a time*—and then to die and get the Hell out of the way of the next generation. We are being asked to give up most of the things that make life worth living—including sovereignty over our own bodies—in exchange for a fantasy of never dying. This transaction deserves perhaps more scrutiny than it has received.

And while I am deeply skeptical of much of what our health services industry does, I can honestly say vaccines were not even on my radar before the covid pandemic. But that has changed, after bearing witness to the stories of people who were so pro-vax they volunteered for the covid vaccine trials—or enrolled their children in these trials—and suffered devastating consequences as a result. I find their stories eminently believable—much more so than the pronouncements of slick paladins on television admonishing us to "follow the science." I have also experienced personally the effects of vaccine injury—which I share with you in the pages that follow.

I have centered this book around five main characters. One is a physician, two are public health researchers, and one is a patient advocate with a long record of speaking truth to power. The fifth is Ron Johnson, the Republican Senator from Wisconsin, seen by some as a polarizing figure. But when the covid-vaccine-injured (most of them Democrats) looked for someone in Congress to champion their cause, he was the only one who stepped forward.

We wrestled with the decision of what to call this work. I suggested *The Clot Shot*, but Dr. Healy pointed out that such a title would never make it past the social media censors. This is more than a bit ironic, given that one of the themes of this book is censorship by social media sites. I also suggested *How the Drug Companies and Government Regulatory Agencies Concealed the Truth about the Covid Vaccines* as a subtitle, but in fact we do not know the full truth about these products and may not know for many years. But we are inviting you to come and sit with our uncertainty for a while, and see what comes of it.

I have not attempted to write the definitive history of the covid pandemic—that is an effort to be left to some future historian, and one that will require many volumes. My intentions here are more modest—to provide the reader with a guidebook to a situation that continues to unfold.

As the kids and I walked back to their house that unseasonably warm November afternoon, it occurred to me that the dystopian science fiction nightmares I used to read as a boy were rapidly becoming today's humdrum reality. The Medical Dictatorship threatens to envelop us all like a dark cloud. I want something better than that for my nephew and nieces. If, in some small way, this book can help light the way to a brighter future for these beautiful children, I shall consider my time on earth to have been well spent.

The covid pandemic has brought out the worst in a lot of people, but it has also brought out the best in some. You are about to meet some members of both groups of people in this work.

CHAPTER ONE

Unleashing
The Power Of Science

December 2019 - January 2021

Nobody Sees This as a Way to Make Billions of Dollars

Sometime in early December of 2019, a man living in Wuhan, a city of some eleven million souls located in Hubei province in China, fell ill with pneumonia of unknown cause. Other, similar cases soon followed. The new illness was characterized by fever, cough, muscle aches and pains, and fatigue, along with (less commonly) headache, diarrhea, and the coughing up of mucus or blood. More than half developed acute respiratory distress syndrome, a condition caused by buildup of fluid in the air sacs of the lungs, resulting in severe shortness of breath.[1]

On the last day of that year, China reported a cluster of cases of pneumonia of unknown etiology to the World Health Organization. By that time, twenty-seven cases of the mysterious ailment had been reported to authorities, but no deaths.[2] Contemporary accounts made a point of noting that many of these cases had contact with what was euphemistically described as a "seafood market," but none of them saw fit to mention that the city of Wuhan is home to a secret bioweapons lab run by a murderous and one of the most secretive and controlling regimes in human history.

On 7 January 2020, Chinese scientists announced they had identified the mysterious infectious agent as one of the coronaviruses, a family of viruses named after the "crown" of club-shaped spikes projecting from the outer surface, which it uses to gain entry into the host cell.[3] Four of these viruses were known to cause common cold symptoms in humans, and two more—SARS-CoV (now known as SARS-CoV-1) and MERS-CoV—had caused large numbers of deaths.[4]

Sixteen days later, the Coalition for Epidemic Preparedness—an organization founded with funding from the Bill and Melinda Gates Foundation along with grant money from the Wellcome Trust and the governments of India and Norway—announced a new partnership with National Institute of Allergies and Infectious Diseases (NIAID, a part of the National Institutes of Health) along with the biotech startup Moderna to speed the development of vaccines against the new pathogen, promising to leverage Moderna's mRNA vaccine platform to "bring a new pathogen from gene sequencing to clinical testing in 16 weeks."[5] The development of a new vaccine is a process which usually is expected to take between ten and fifteen years.

That same day, an article in *Business Insider India* reported that Moderna had signed a contract with the National Institutes of Health stating that any mRNA vaccines developed by the joint venture would be the property of both organizations. The piece went on to quote NIH Director Francis Collins:

> Talking to the companies, I don't hear any of them say they think this [vaccine] is a money-maker. I think they want to recoup their costs and maybe make a tiny percentage of increase over that.
>
> Nobody sees this as a way to make billions of dollars.[6]

On 11 February, the Coronavirus Study Group gave the new virus a name: SARS-CoV-2, a contraction of Sudden Acute Respiratory Syndrome Coronavirus 2.[7] That same day, the World Health Organization Director-General announced that the illness caused by this infectious agent would henceforth be known COVID-19, a contraction of Coronavirus Disease 2019. By that time, there were 42,708 confirmed cases in China and 1,017 deaths. Outside of China there were 393 cases in twenty-four countries and one reported death.[8]

Your Single Source of Truth

For each one of us on what former *New York Times* reporter Alex Berenson would later come to refer to as "Team Reality,"[9] there came a defining moment in the pandemic when we realized this was not about any of the things we were told us it was. For me that moment came early, in March of 2020, when the epicenter of the pandemic shifted from China to the Po Valley in Italy—an area with a chronically underfunded health care system and some of the worst air pollution in Europe. News accounts informed us that the average patient there dying of the coronavirus was seventy-eight years old, with three or more complicating conditions, and I remember thinking to myself *Wait a minute—then the sky is not falling, after all.*

Nonetheless, it was right after that that the institutions where I taught switched to remote learning, while the populace chafed under a mélange of ever-shifting nonsensical restrictions, the likes of which had never been seen in the peacetime history of this or any other country. Schools were closed, millions of workers were told they were not "essential," and the masks served as an omnipresent grim reminder of the specter of death supposedly stalking us all.

For my part, I did not suffer unduly. I had the luxury of continuing to work at home, and I found I disliked remote instruction less than I had thought I would. I certainly did not miss spending eight or more hours a week freeway flying between my various teaching jobs. I got lots of writing done, and I ramped up the walking to ten miles a day.

Not everyone was as fortunate. Joblessness, homelessness, alcohol consumption, depression, substance abuse, suicidal ideation, and prescriptions for antidepressants all skyrocketed in the wake of pandemic restrictions.[10]

On 22 March, the World Health Organization Scientific Advisory Group for Emergencies (SAGE) issued a secret report titled "Options for Increasing Adherence to Social Distancing Measures,"[11] which contained these ominous words:

> A substantial number of people still do not feel sufficiently personally threatened.

There was nothing at all in the report about engaging with citizens as intelligent, self-governing women and men with facts and data. Instead, the psy-ops experts (aka "the SAGE Behavioural Science Sub-Group") recommended fear ("hard-hitting emotional messaging"), guilt ("responsibility to others"), and scapegoating ("social approval").

As the death toll mounted, rumors began to fly. Fortunately, government officials and the media stood ready to help out. On 28 February, a piece in *Vice* put to rest irrational fears that the government would ever force people to get a vaccine for the coronavirus,[12] and at a press conference on 19 March, New Zealand Prime Minister Jacinda Ardern fielded a reporter's question about a "viral hoax" that a lockdown was imminent in New Zealand, replying "That's the kind of thing that adds to the anxiety that people feel."[13] At the same presser, the Prime Minister offered these now-famous words of reassurance:

> Dismiss anything else. We will continue to be your single source of truth.

Six days after that, New Zealand went into lockdown.[14]

Warp Speed

Meanwhile, three days before Prime Minister Ardern made her announcement, NIAID announced that Phase I trials of the new vaccine it had produced in collaboration with Moderna had begun. This product, dubbed mRNA-1273, contained the messenger RNA sequence for the coronavirus spike protein, which was intended to force the body's cells to manufacture that molecule, in hopes of generating a robust immune response.[15] The day the announcement was made, Moderna's stock price jumped twenty-four percent, closing at $26.49.[16]

Exactly one month later, Moderna announced it had received a $483 million contract from the Biomedical Advanced Research and Development Authority (BARDA) to accelerate the development of its new vaccine.[17]

As of 1 May, cumulative reported covid deaths had reached 61,000 for the US and 236,000 worldwide. On the seventh of that month, Pfizer announced it would begin human trials of its new vaccine, dubbed BNT162b2, which it developed in collaboration with the German firm BioNTech and which employs the same type of RNA platform as Moderna.[18] Eight days later, at a Rose Garden Ceremony, President Trump introduced Project Warp Speed to facilitate the development of covid vaccines as well as the scaling up of manufacturing systems to deliver hundreds of millions or even billions of doses as quickly as possible. The project was jointly headed by Four-Star General Gustave Perna and Moncef Slaoui, former head of Research and Development at GlaxoSmithKline and current Moderna board member. Dr. Slaoui stepped down from the Moderna Board of Directors but retained millions of dollars' worth of stock in the company.[19]

Following Dr. Slaoui's appointment, Massachusetts Senator Elizabeth Warren tweeted that it was a "huge conflict of interest" for him to hold on to his Moderna stock, which jumped in value from $10 million to $12.4 million immediately after Project Warp Speed was unveiled. In a tweet that was later deleted, Slaoui replied "There is no conflict of interest, and never has been," but subsequently relented, promising to sell his Moderna shares and donate the excess profits to cancer research.[20]

The race was on.

No one seems to have noticed at the time that by pouring billions of dollars into manufacturing systems for shots that had not even been trialed, they were creating an enterprise that was too big to fail.

Safe and Effective

On 12 June, Reuters informed its readers that "A series of studies in mice of Moderna Inc's COVID-19 [vaccine] lent some assurance that it may not increase the risk of more severe disease, and that one dose may provide protection against the novel coronavirus, according to preliminary data released on Friday."[21]

On 22 July, the United States Department of Defense and the Department of Health and Human Services announced they had entered into a joint agreement to pay Pfizer $1.95 billion to provide 100 million doses of its vaccine, with the ability to acquire up to 500 million additional doses.[22]

Five days later, Phase III trials for both the Moderna vaccine and the Pfizer vaccine began. Both products were to be administered in the form of two intramuscular injections, twenty-one days apart in the case of the Pfizer shot, which contained thirty micrograms of RNA, and twenty-eight days for the Moderna product, which contained one hundred micrograms. The primary endpoint for both trials was covid infection of any severity, occurring at least seven days after the second dose of the Pfizer shot, or fourteen days after the second dose of the Moderna vax.

On 18 August, FDA Commissioner Stephen Hahn and two other prominent officials of that agency authored a piece in *Health Affairs* intended to reassure the public that any covid vaccines would be safe and effective. The three experts had this to say:

Given that recent polling indicates evidence of vaccine hesitancy among Americans for COVID-19, it is also necessary for public health officials to offer reassurance that any potential vaccine will be safe and effective.

First, the agency established clear recommendations for vaccine performance prior to the initiation of Phase III trials to provide assurance that any authorized vaccine will meet appropriate standards for safety and effectiveness.

Second, FDA has committed to use an advisory committee composed of independent experts to ensure deliberations about authorization or licensure are transparent for the public.

In this blog we will clarify ongoing government activities for a COVID-19 vaccine and detail the steps FDA has taken to ensure the safety and effectiveness of a potential vaccine.

First, it recommends clinical trials for COVID-19 vaccines be sufficiently powered to demonstrate meaningful effects for the intended population. Given that the virus has disproportionately affected specific populations (e.g., racial minorities, elderly adults, individuals with comorbidities) sponsors should ensure that study populations include adequate representation from these groups.

Second, the guidance recommends that sponsors follow best practices for clinical research, with FDA recommending the use of randomized, double-blinded, and placebo-controlled study designs.

Third, FDA provides recommendations for the safety and effectiveness of a COVID-19 vaccine. The agency recommends that sponsors use placebo-controlled randomized trials to test vaccine candidates which, to be considered effective, should prevent COVID-19 in at least 50% of patients.[23]

Standing with Science

Not everyone was so sanguine about all this. On 24 August, an essay in the *BMJ* raised concerns about the advisability of recommending the COVID-19 vaccines without full clinical trial data being made publicly available.[24] The piece was authored by two prominent critics of the pharmaceutical industry: Peter Doshi and David Healy.

Dr. Doshi is a Professor of Pharmaceutical Health Services Research at the University of Maryland. Dr. Healy is a psychiatrist and the author of *Pharmageddon*.[25] For most of his career he was Clinical Professor of Psychiatry at Bangor University in Wales, but just recently he switched his base of operations to the Department of Family Medicine at McMaster University in Ontario. In June of 2013, both men (along with several co-authors) published a paper in the *BMJ* titled "Restoring Invisible and Abandoned Trials: A Call for People to Publish the Findings"[26] in which they stated they had 178,000 pages of previously confidential drug company documents pertaining to clinical trials which either never had been published or which had been misreported. They called upon the sponsors of these trials to publish the unpublished studies, and formally correct or retract the misreported ones. They further stated that if the sponsors failed to do so, the data would be considered "public access data" which others would be allowed to publish.

The article amounted to a manifesto demanding a new era of clinical trial transparency, and led directly to the re-analysis by Dr. Healy and others of GlaxoSmithKline's infamous Study 329, which had reported that Paxil was safe and effective for treating major depression in adolescents, even though the re-analysis of company's own data showed no difference between the active drug and placebo for any of eight original outcome variables, and that one out of eight children getting Paxil suffered from suicidality or self-harm.[27] In plain English, the stuff was totally ineffective and drove the kids crazy to boot. Now the two men were turning their attention to the covid vaccine trials.

"Data transparency builds the foundation for information we can trust," the two researchers wrote. "Data secrecy, by contrast, creates risks too large to take." They went on to point out the two risks of not making data transparent: Overestimation of the benefits of a medicine, and underestimation of the harms.

> Only open data can allow other researchers with the ability to analyze it to do so, generating the trust that stems from knowing that judgements have been scrutinized and challenged. Data transparency also creates the optimal environment for products—and there will be many covid-19 products, to be sure—to compete on the strength of their evidence base, not on the strength of promotion and buzz.[28]

The two experts concluded by calling on doctors and professional societies to refuse, in the absence of data transparency, to endorse COVID-19 products as based on science. In the Declaration of Competing Interests, Dr. Healy added that he would review the options for a legal challenge to any attempt to force him to take any vaccine whose data are not fully available.

On 8 September, the CEO's of nine pharmaceutical companies, including Pfizer, BioNTech, Moderna, as well as six others involved in vaccine research, signed a pledge to "Stand with science" and "Make the safety and well-being of vaccinated individuals the top priority of the first COVID-19 vaccines." They also pledged to submit covid vaccines for approval only after "demonstrating safety and efficacy through a Phase 3 clinical study that is designed and conducted to meet requirements of expert regulatory authorities such as the FDA."[29]

The document made no mention of data transparency, nor did it mention that "expert regulatory authorities such as the FDA" are funded, in a large measure, through drug company "user fees."

The next day, Eric Topol, Editor-in-Chief of Medscape and Professor of Molecular Medicine at the Scripps Research Institute, interviewed Paul Offit, Director of the Vaccine Education Center at Children's Hospital in Philadelphia and Professor of Vaccinology at the University of Pennsylvania School of Medicine, for Medscape.[30] The two experts discussed the drugmakers' criteria for a "positive event" in the covid vaccine trials:

> ERIC TOPOL: And to clarify, because this is important, we're not talking about just a PCR-positive mild infection. It has to be moderate to severe illness to qualify as an event, correct?
>
> PAUL OFFIT: That's right.

Five days later an article in the *New York Times* argued that the lack of data transparency is unacceptable, given that the federal government had cut billion-dollar deals with each of the nine companies that had signed the pledge. The piece went on to quote Saad B. Omer, director of the Yale Institute for Global Health, as follows: "Look we paid for [the data]. So it's reasonable to ask for it."[31]

Four days after that, another *NYT* article reported that both Pfizer and Moderna had agreed to make the trial protocols publicly available, an unprecedented move.[32]

"I want to acknowledge a good deed done," the article quoted Dr. Doshi as saying. "They have opened up, for the first time, the ability of researchers not involved in the trial to form their own independent judgement about the design of the study."[33]

A Key Secondary Endpoint

As it turned out, the release of the trial protocols raised new concerns. In a 21 October article in the *BMJ*, Dr. Doshi explained that while most people probably would assume that dubbing a vaccine "effective" meant that it prevented deaths, hospitalizations, serious illness, transmission, or some other clinically relevant endpoint, in fact the Phase III trials were not powered to do so—despite official assurances to the contrary. The primary endpoint was covid infection of any severity. A cough plus a positive antibody test would be enough to qualify.[34] This is an endpoint of dubious value, given that the vast majority of covid cases resolve themselves in a short period of time with no lingering after-effects.

This was a point the drugmakers and their allies did not seem interested in making clear to the public. In a press release, Moderna had misleadingly told the public that hospital admissions were a "key secondary endpoint"—neglecting to mention that a secondary endpoint is one a trial is not powered to measure. And the National Institutes of Health had employed a similar rhetorical sleight of hand, informing readers that "the trial also aims to study whether the vaccine can prevent severe COVID-19" and "the trial also seeks to answer if the vaccine can prevent death caused by COVID-19," again without mentioning that the trial was not powered to answer either of these questions.[35]

Moreover, the references to "severe COVID-19" and "deaths caused by COVID-19" were red herrings, begging the question of whether the vaccine reduces the frequency of all deaths or all serious adverse events.

The article went on to quote Moderna Chief Medical Office Tal Zaks at length:

> The trial is precluded from judging [hospital admissions], based on what is a reasonable size and duration to serve the public good here.
>
> Would I like to know that this [vaccine] prevents mortality? Sure, because I believe it does. I just don't think it's feasible within the timeframe [of the trial]—too many would die waiting for the results before we ever knew that.
>
> Our trial will not demonstrate prevention of transmission, because in order to do that you have to swab people

twice a week for long periods, and that becomes operationally untenable.

A 30,000 [participant] trial is already a fairly large trial. If you're asking for a 300,000 [participant] trial then you need to talk to the people who are paying for it, because now you're talking about not a $500m to $1bn trials, you're talking about something 10 times the size.

So what is the public good being served if hundreds of millions or even billions of people are enticed or coerced into taking the vaccine without any trial data showing it reduced the likelihood of any clinically relevant outcome? Dr. Zaks had two answers for that question. In the first place, he argued, we do have a bad outcome as an endpoint—COVID-19 disease. In the second place, he claimed that influenza vaccines protect against severe illness better than they do against mild illness, and therefore if the covid vaccine prevents mild covid infection we may assume it must protect against severe infection, as well.[36] This is as blatant an example of the fallacy of inclusion as one could hope to find.

In fact, as Dr. Doshi pointed out, after decades of administering flu shots, there still is no convincing evidence that these preparations "save lives."[37] Only two placebo-controlled trials have ever been performed, and neither was powered to detect an effect on hospital admissions or deaths. Moreover, a 2005 study had shown no correlation between increased vaccination in elderly people and all-cause winter mortality.[38]

Dr. Doshi went on to note that history shows many examples of serious adverse events from vaccines that were hastily brought on to the market, including cases of contaminated polio vaccines in 1955, Guillain-Barré syndrome caused by influenza vaccines in 1976, and narcolepsy caused by influenza vaccines in 2009. He further noted that the covid vaccines trials were not powered to detect rare but serious adverse events.

Finally, Dr. Doshi pointed out that children, pregnant or breast-feeding women, and the immunocompromised were excluded from the trials, and while some elderly people were enrolled, the trials were not powered to demonstrate a benefit in this vulnerable population—again, in spite of official assurances to the contrary.

All of these words of caution fell upon deaf ears.

Science Will Win

On 9 November, Pfizer announced in a press release that their new vaccine was "more than 90% effective in preventing COVID-19 in participants without prior evidence of SARS-CoV-2 infection." The press release also quoted Pfizer CEO Albert Bourla as follows: "Today is a great day for science and humanity."[39]

That same day, in an interview with *Axios*, Dr. Bourla explained his decision not to accept funding from Operation Warp Speed:

> The reason I did that was to liberate our scientists.
>
> And with that I unleashed the power of science.
>
> I'm very happy that we made this decision, because we had the results I think much faster than otherwise if we were not unencumbered.
>
> I didn't take money, not only from the US government, but then the other government in the world that they were offering.[40]

Seven days later, Moderna issued a press release claiming their product was "94.5% effective." The statement quoted Moderna CEO Stéphane Bancel, who noted: "This is a pivotal moment in the development of our COVID-19 vaccine candidate" and went on to thank the National Institute for Allergies and Infectious Disease as well as "our partners at BARDA and Operation Warp Speed, who have been instrumental in accelerating our progress to this point."[41]

Amidst this chorus of self-praise there were a few dissenting voices. On 23 November the venerable journal *Nature* reported that Pfizer had sent a letter dated 10 November to trial participants stating the company was already exploring ways to offer the shot to patients enrolled in the placebo arm of the trial—and so beginning the process of eliminating the control group.[42] And just three days later, in a piece in *BMJ Blogs*, Dr. Doshi pointed out that Pfizer's and Moderna's claims of over ninety percent effectiveness for the primary endpoint, covid infection of any severity, were based on relative risk, not absolute risk.[43] This is a metric which can vastly over-inflate the seeming effectiveness of a product.

The Pfizer trial enrolled forty-four thousand subjects, split equally between the treatment and placebo arms. Pfizer recorded 162 cases of covid in the placebo group versus eight in the treatment group. In other words, out of 141 patients who took the shot, there would have been one fewer case. When you put it in those terms, it doesn't seem nearly as impressive.

The Moderna trial enrolled thirty thousand subjects, again split equally between the placebo and treatment groups. In this case there were ninety-five cases of covid in the placebo arm, versus five in the treatment arm. This works out to an even more paltry one in 161 reduction in risk.

These four numbers—162 cases versus eight, and ninety-five cases versus five—have formed the basis for injecting hundreds of millions of people worldwide with a type of experimental gene therapy never before deployed in the general population.

More disturbingly, the trial protocols for both companies seemed to include instructions to clinicians to guess who was getting the active treatment and who was not.

This is the language copied and pasted from the Pfizer protocol:

> During the 7 days following each vaccination, potential COVID-19 symptoms that overlap with solicited systemic events (i.e., fever, chills, new or increased muscle pain, diarrhea, vomiting) should ***not*** trigger a potential COVID-19 illness visit unless, in the investigator's opinion, the clinical

picture is more indicative of a possible COVID-19 illness than vaccine reactogenicity. [Emphasis added.][44]

Here is the comparable language copied and pasted from the Moderna protocol:

It is important to note that some of the symptoms of COVID-19 overlap with solicited systemic ARs that are expected after vaccination with mRNA-1273 (eg, myalgia, headache, fever, and chills). During the first 7 days after vaccination, when these solicited ARs are common, investigators should use their clinical judgement to decide if an NP swab should be collected.[45]

This is a blatant violation of the fundamental principle of double-blind clinical trials, which is that neither clinicians nor patients should be aware of which ones are getting the active treatment and which are getting placebo.

Again Dr. Doshi reiterated that the trials were not powered to detect whether the vaccine lowered the death rate, or the rate of transmission, or the rate of covid infection in important subgroups such as the frail elderly. There were no data available at all three months, six months, or twelve months after the shot. Furthermore, children, adolescents, and the immunocompromised were largely excluded from the trials.[46]

Again, all of these words of caution fell upon deaf ears.

In addition, while some participants with prior history of covid infection were included in the trials, covid cases (not to mention serious adverse events, including death) in this group were not counted *as a separate endpoint.*

On 10 December, the FDA Vaccines and Related Biological Products Advisory Committee (VRBPAC) voted seventeen-to-four (with one abstention) to authorize the Pfizer shot for emergency use. An Emergency Use Authorization allows a product to be used in an emergency to diagnose, treat, or prevent life-threatening diseases when there are no adequate, approved, available alternatives.

This decision was announced by the FDA in a press release the following day, which contained this disclaimer:

> At this time, data are not available to make a determination about how long the vaccine will provide protection, nor is there evidence that the vaccine prevents transmission of SARS-CoV-2 from person to person.[47]

In the excitement, these words of caution went almost unnoticed. That same day, Dr. Bourla exulted:

> Pfizer's purpose is breakthroughs that change patients' lives, and in our 171-year history there has never been a more urgent need for a breakthrough than today.
>
> As a US company, today's news brings great pride and tremendous joy that Pfizer has risen to the challenge to develop a vaccine that has the potential to bring an end to this devastating pandemic. We have worked tirelessly to make the impossible possible, steadfast in our belief that science will win.[48]

His enthusiasm was not shared by everybody. During the public response section of the VRBPAC meeting, patient advocate Kim Witczak had this to say:

> The only ones who have 100% immunity in this are the pharma companies. They get all the benefits of sales without any legal liability should something go wrong.[49]

Kim has experience with Pfizer's products. Seventeen years earlier, her husband Woody was prescribed Pfizer's blockbuster drug Zoloft for insomnia. Shortly after he began taking the drug, Woody, who had no history of depression or suicidality, went into the garage and hanged himself. He was thirty-seven years old.

Shifting the Goalposts

On 12 December, the European Medicines Agency granted conditional authorization for the Pfizer shot,[50] now christened with the tongue-twisting moniker Comirnaty—a mish-mosh of the words COVID-19, mRNA, community, and immunity. This new brand name had beat out such worthy contenders as Covuity, RnaxCovi, and Kovimerna.

Six days later, the FDA authorized the Moderna shot, later to be christened Spikevax, for emergency use.

That same day, a piece by the BBC noted that Moderna had received $2.6 billion in government funding to develop its vaccine, and that Pfizer, Dr. Bourla's proclamations notwithstanding, had received in excess of $270 million.[51]

Six days after that, an article in the *New York Times* noted that NIAID Director Anthony Fauci had been playing fast and loose with his estimates of the degree of vaccine coverage needed to attain herd immunity against the coronavirus.[52] "Herd immunity" is a concept originally developed by veterinary scientists to enable them to understand the spread of disease in, well, herds. It means simply the ability of a population of animals to resist the spread of infectious disease. The term was introduced in 1918, in a bulletin produced by the Kansas State Agricultural College Experimental Station regarding epidemics of spontaneous miscarriage in assemblages of cattle:

> Abortion disease may be likened to a fire, which, if new fuel is not constantly added, soon dies down. Herd immunity is developed, therefore, by retaining the immune cows, raising the calves, and avoiding the introduction of foreign cattle.[53]

William Topley and Graham Wilson, authors of *Principles of Bacteriology and Immunity* (which served as the canonical textbook of medical microbiology for decades), extended the concept to mice, in their studies of the spread of epidemics in caged populations of these animals.[54] Surgeon Captain Sheldon Dudley, Professor at the Royal Naval College, was the first to apply the concept to human beings, in regard to outbreaks of diphtheria at the Greenwich Naval School for boys.[55] He noted that herd immunity is a function not just of the proportion of members of a population immune to a given disease, but also the spatial relations of individuals in the population to one another as well as nutritional status of the individuals, the infectivity of the pathogen, and probably a whole host of other factors as well.[56]

Herd immunity is a heuristic construct, not something that can be measured. Early models predicted that herd immunity was reached only when a high threshold of individual immunity was reached—as high as ninety percent in some models—but these models assumed contact between members of the population was random. That may be a reasonable approximation when we are talking about herds of cattle in pens or mice in cages, but it is an absolutely indefensible assumption when applied to human society. More recent models set the value needed for herd immunity much lower—as low as ten percent in some cases—but no one really knows.

None of this stopped Dr. Fauci in successive interviews with the media from progressively raising the bid from "sixty to seventy percent" to "seventy, seventy-five percent" to "seventy-five, eighty, eighty-five percent." In a telephone interview, the NIAID Director stated he believed that the true figure was closer to ninety percent, and that he had been moving the goalposts slowly and deliberately, so as not to discourage the public from getting the shot by having them think the goal of herd immunity was unattainable.

This was a disturbing line of reasoning, for three reasons. In the first place, Dr. Fauci seemed to be indicating a willingness to engage in falsehoods in pursuit of some imagined "greater good." In the second place, he seemed to be admitting that the individual benefit-to-cost ratio was not enough to tip the balance in favor of getting the vaccine. Perhaps most disturbingly, he seemed to be deliberately confusing *herd immunity* with *vaccine coverage*—and in the process ignoring the reality of natural immunity, something as well-established as the Law of Gravity or the Periodic Table in chemistry.

The mendacity went beyond a few casual remarks in interviews. Four days after the *NYT* piece ran, Jeffrey Tucker, then Editorial Director for the American Institute for Economic Research, revealed that the World Health Organization had quietly changed its definition of "herd immunity" on its website.[57] The former definition, archived on 9 June 2020, was as follows:

> Herd immunity is protection from an infectious disease that happens when a population is immune either through vacci-nation or immunity developed through previous infection.

But in a screenshot dated 13 November 2020, the definition had been changed so as to ignore the reality of naturally acquired immunity—as if only vaccine-enforced immunity counted:

> 'Herd immunity,' also known as 'population immunity,' is a concept used for vaccination, in which a population can be protected from a certain virus if a threshold of vaccination is reached. Herd immunity is achieved by protecting people from a virus, not by exposing them to it.

No explanation was offered for the change.

In a blistering commentary, Tucker wrote:

> In effect, this change at WHO ignores and even wipes out 100 years of medical advances in virology, immunology, and epidemiology. It is thoroughly unscientific—shilling for

the vaccine industry in exactly the same way the conspiracy theorists say that WHO has been doing since the beginning of the pandemic.

Now the "science" is actually deleting its own history, airbrushing over what it used to know and replacing it with something misleading at best and patently false at worst.

On the last day of the year, the results of the Pfizer Phase III trial were published in the *New England Journal of Medicine*.[58] Of the twenty-nine authors, eighteen were employees of Pfizer and held stock in that company.[59]

By this time, the coronavirus pandemic had claimed a reported 356,000 lives in the United States and 1.9 million worldwide.

Protocol Violations

In another piece in *BMJ Blogs* appearing 4 January 2021, Dr. Doshi reiterated his concerns and added some new ones.[60] By this time journal reports for the Phase III trials for both the Pfizer shot and the Moderna product were available, along with 400 pages of summary data presented by and to the FDA.

Dr. Doshi pointed out that according to the FDA briefing document, the incidence of "suspected COVID-19" (covid-like symptoms not confirmed by a PCR test) in the Pfizer trial was similar in both arms of the trial: out of a total of 3,410 such cases, there were 1,594 occurring in the treatment arm and 1,816 among participants given placebo. These figures include 696 cases occurring within seven days after either of the two doses. The preponderance of those occurred in the treatment arm—409 cases, as opposed to 287 in the placebo arm

Since the presentation of "suspected covid" is essentially the same as that of confirmed covid, Dr. Doshi argued that the efficacy of the vaccine against developing covid-like symptoms was a paltry nineteen percent—far below the ninety percent efficacy figure trumpeted by Pfizer.

What's more, the FDA review of the Pfizer vaccine noted that 371 patients were dropped from the trial for "protocol violations." Most of these—311 to be exact—were in the treatment arm. By contrast, only thirty-six patients were dropped from the Moderna trial for protocol violations—twelve in the treatment group and twenty-four in the placebo group. Why were so many patients dropped from the Pfizer trial, and why the vast discrepancy between the treatment and placebo groups? No one was saying.

Dr. Doshi went on to mention that, while four independent university-affiliated physicians had adjudicated the primary events in the Moderna trial, Pfizer had left that task to three Pfizer employees.

Dr. Doshi wound up by noting that the raw trial data still was not available, although the Pfizer protocol said the data would be made available twenty-four months after the completion of the study, while Moderna's data sharing statement said data "may" be made available "upon request" once the trial is complete, which would translate to sometime in mid-to-late 2022, since the trial was planned to last for two years.

Once again, all of these words of caution fell upon deaf ears.

The Highest Standards and Traditions of Science

The same day Dr. Doshi's piece appeared, the World Health Organization quietly changed its definition of herd immunity back to the one accepted by science for decades. Once again no announcement was made, nor was any explanation offered.[61]

One week later, Dr. Healy published an appeal in his blog at RxISK.org, asking readers to submit reports of covid vaccine injuries, along with these comments:

On drug labels, there is a section for other reports which most clinical staff and likely most of the rest of us read as reports sent in by Flat-Earthers and anti-vaxxers. We see companies as being wonderfully transparent including even these in the label and of course we are not going to believe that these things are caused by a drug or a vaccine.

In fact, hazards only get into this section when companies have done their damnedest to explain an event away. Left with only one option that their drug has likely caused it, they include mention in this part of their label.

My children are frontline healthcare workers one of whom has had a covid vaccine and the other will take.

I have painted myself into a corner in a BMJ contribution with Peter Doshi about data transparency, where I declared under the conflict of interest heading an unwillingness to take a vaccine where there was not access to the underlying data. This position is not anti-vaccine any more than it is anti-medication—I make my living prescribing meds. It's anti-sequestration of data.[62]

Four days after that, Dr. Doshi's piece in *BMJ Blogs* was the target of a blog post by David Gorski, Professor of Surgery and Oncology at Wayne State University School of Medicine and Managing Editor of Science-Based Medicine. The post was titled "Why Is Peter Doshi Still an editor at the BMJ?"[63]

Dr. Gorski took Dr. Doshi to task for the nineteen percent efficacy figure, stating "It is just not reasonable to just assume that all cases of respiratory illness in a sample of 30,000 people are due to COVID-19." But that was not Doshi's argument. His argument was this: what difference does it make if people get the shot to avoid covid but have an almost equal chance of developing another illness with the same clinical presentation? That's a serious question, and it deserves a serious answer, but Gorski does not provide us with one.

Dr. Gorski also blasted Dr. Doshi for calling attention to the fact that 371 patients were excluded from the Pfizer trial for protocol violations:

> Most clinical trialists would be **thrilled** to have **only** 0.5% of the subjects in one of their trials need to be excluded from the final analysis for protocol deviations, and even given the imbalance in deviations between the placebo and vaccine groups this is a number too small to have significantly affected the final analysis. [Emphasis in the original]

This is an astonishing statement. To be sure, the one in two hundred figure seems tiny, but so is the reported one in 141 reduction in absolute risk of symptomatic covid in the treatment arm. Dr. Gorski's argument begs the question of why such a hugely disproportionate number of patients (311 versus sixty) were excluded from the treatment arm. How many rare but serious adverse events were concealed among those 311 patients? If Gorski has any idea, he isn't saying.

Dr. Gorski goes on to slam Dr. Doshi for "implying nefariousness by pointing out that the event adjudication committee for the Pfizer trial consisted of three Pfizer employees"—as if questioning the integrity of a multibillion-dollar drug company should put Doshi beyond the pale. Given Pfizer's track record,[64] that argument seems questionable, to say the least.

Indeed, coming as it did from the managing editor of an organization that plumes itself for its "dedication to evaluating medical treatments and products of interest to the public in a scientific light, and promoting the highest standards and traditions of science in health care,"[65] the piece was light on facts and heavy on invective and sophomoric attempts at humor. Some selections follow:

While all the while claiming he's not "antivaccine," [Dr. Doshi] has parroted more than a few antivaccine talking points himself.

Periodically he publishes posts for The BMJ that are—to put it kindly—far below the standards that a medical journal with the history of The BMJ should ever associate itself with.

"Bad science" is Peter Doshi's middle name, actually, going all the way back at least to 2006, accelerating in 2009 as the H1N1 influenza pandemic hit, and continuing all the way to 2021. It's his schtick. It's what he's known for.

Is he "just asking questions," a.k.a. JAQing off?

The piece was illustrated with a large color photograph of Dr. Doshi, captioned "Peter Doshi, trying to look academic."

On 19 January, the financial and investment company Finaria reported that Pfizer-BioNTech and Moderna were expected to earn $14.7 billion in vaccine sales by 2023.[66]

The next day, Stephan Hahn stepped down from his position as FDA commissioner, to be replaced with Janet Woodcock, former Acting Director of the FDA's Center for Drug Evaluation and Research.[67]

Five days after that, the CDC urged everyone to get vaccinated for the covid regardless of previous infection, noting that "natural immunity varies from person to person" and "experts do not yet know how long someone is protected [by natural immunity]."[68]

Coming as it did barely a month into the vaccine rollout, the hollowness of this argument should have been immediately apparent to all.

By the last day of January, total reported covid deaths topped 455,000 in the United States and 2.3 million worldwide.

* * *

In summary: the Pfizer-BioNTech and Moderna products were rushed into emergency use based on trials with a non-clinically-relevant primary endpoint, no access to the patient-level data, potential unblinding problems (encouraging clinicians to guess which patients had been given the active treatment and which had not), an excess of patients dropped from the treatment arm of the Pfizer trial for unspecified "protocol violations," and not even the drugmakers claiming their own data could demonstrate these products reduced the rate of death, or serious adverse events, or hospitalizations, or intubations, or transmission, or any other clinically relevant endpoint.

But this story was just beginning.

CHAPTER TWO

How Covid Kills, How the Vax Works, and How the Vax May Kill

How Covid Kills

Now is a good time to step back and review the science behind the coronavirus and the "vaccines" being touted as the remedy for the pandemic.

As far as science is concerned, every living thing, from the smallest microbe to the mightiest of the great whales, is nothing more than a temporary vessel built to contain genetic information. This information is stored in the sequence of nucleoside bases which make up DNA, which is transcribed to messenger RNA (mRNA). Little nanomachines called ribosomes in turn translate information encoded in mRNA into the sequence of amino acids which make up proteins.

There are twenty different kinds of amino acids found in proteins. Each protein consists of a chain of anywhere from several dozen to several thousand of these amino acids, strung together in a specific sequence. All complex biological molecules either are proteins, or else they are manufactured by enzymes, which themselves are proteins. So proteins are the building blocks of living things.

Whether or not a virus qualifies as a "living thing" is a matter of semantics, but it is indisputable that a virus is simpler than the simplest living cell. By itself a virus is an inert lump of matter, incapable of harnessing or using energy, replicating or transcribing genetic information, or manufacturing protein. Indeed, viruses can be crystallized, a property we do not normally associate with living things.

A virus consists of nothing more than a strand of genetic material, either DNA or RNA, surrounded by a protein capsule. Some viruses wear a cloak of phospholipid bilayer, but this cloak was purloined from the host cell from which it sprang, not made by the virus.

The virus invades a host cell and hijacks the machinery of that cell to make multiple copies of the viral genome. Information in the viral genome is then transcribed to viral mRNA, which in turn is translated into viral proteins. The viral genomes and the viral proteins spontaneously self-assemble to make new virus particles, or virions, and then the host cell bursts and dies, releasing a cohort of new virions which can invade more host cells.

We have already noted that SARS-CoV-2 belongs to a family of viruses called the coronaviruses. The coronavirus comes wrapped in a membrane which is mainly stolen from the host cell, although this membrane contains viral proteins as well. These viruses store genetic information as a single strand of RNA, arbitrarily designated as (+) RNA because its sequence is identical to that of the messenger RNA. After the virus becomes attached to the host cell, it injects this strand of RNA into the fluid inside the cell, and the host cell's machinery is used to make a complementary strand of (-) RNA, which is then used as a template for the synthesis of more (+) RNA, which in turn is used to direct the synthesis of the coronavirus proteins, including the spike protein.

The virus gains entry into the host cell by means of this spike protein. A host cell membrane protein known as Angiotensin-Converting Enzyme 2, or ACE2, serves as the enzyme which cleaves the spike protein into two subunits, known simply as S1 and S2. S1 binds to ACE2, while S2 directs the fusion of host and viral membranes. In the process, ACE2 is shed by the host cell and so is made unavailable to perform its normal functions. Most of the pernicious effects of the coronavirus are mediated by the disruption of the functioning of this enzyme, so an understanding of how ACE2 works is essential to understanding how the coronavirus does its dirty work, how the vax works, and how the vax may kill.

ACE2 is part of the renin-angiotensin-aldosterone system (RAAS), which regulates blood pressure and salt and water balance. The liver produces the precursor hormone angiotensinogen, a chain of 485 amino acids. The enzyme renin chops off the tail end of Angiotensinogen to form a chain of ten amino acids called Angiotensin I, which can enter one of two pathways.

In the first pathway, which is activated in response to a drop in blood pressure or blood volume, the Angiotensin Converting Enzyme (ACE) located in the cell membrane surface snips the last amino acid off Angiotensin I to form a chain of nine amino acids called Angiotensin II, which binds to the Angiotensin receptors AT1 and AT2. This causes the blood vessels to narrow, and also promotes water resorption by the kidneys. Both of these actions serve to raise blood pressure.

Angiotensin II also promotes blood clotting, inflammation, cell proliferation, cell migration, deposition of fibrous connective tissue (fibrosis), and formation of new blood vessels (angiogenesis). In addition it inhibits wound healing, and promotes the formation of reactive oxygen species along with cell injury and death. All of these are part of the normal response to injury but, left unchecked, can wreak havoc on the body.

The check in this case is provided by the above-mentioned ACE2. This enzyme promotes the conversion of both Angiotensin I and Angiotensin II to a chain of seven amino acids called Angiotensin (1-7). This hormone binds to a cell receptor called MAS/G, and its effects are opposite to those of Angiotensin II: it lowers blood pressure, inhibits clotting, cell proliferation, cell migration, fibrosis, and angiogenesis, and protects against cell injury and death.

ACE2 is most strongly expressed in the endothelial cells that line the smallest blood vessels, or capillaries, as well as the air sacs (alveoli) of the lungs. The downregulation of this enzyme (and the accompanying upregulation of ACE) lead to cell death, fibrosis, thickening of the walls of the alveoli, and a buildup of fluid, pus, and dead cells called lung opacity. What's more, the blood clots that form in response to the spike protein can become dislodged, blocking vessels that supply blood to the lungs—a condition known as pulmonary embolism. All this inhibits the uptake of oxygen, leading to acute respiratory distress syndrome.

The lungs are the organs most affected by COVID-19, but the devastation wrought by the spike protein doesn't end there. ACE2 is expressed not just in the lungs but in other capillary-rich tissues as well, including the brain, the eyes, the heart, the gastrointestinal tract, the liver, the kidneys, the testes, and the subcutaneous fat. The inactivation of this enzyme by the spike protein leads to a variety of toxic effects:

- Neurological: Ischemic strokes, seizures, confusion, migraine, anosmia (loss of sense of smell), ageusia (loss of sense of taste)

- Cardiac: Pericarditis (inflammation of the membrane that surrounds the heart), myocarditis (inflammation of the heart muscle itself), cardiac arrythmia, heart attacks

- Hepatic: Elevated levels of enzymes indicating liver failure

- Renal: Acute kidney injury

These effects can feed off one another. Lack of oxygen (hypoxia) and kidney failure both can lead to metabolic acidosis, which in turn causes decreased cardiac output, cardiac arrythmia, muscle wasting, bone loss, etc. Decreased cardiac output contributes to hypoxia, while cardiac arrythmia increases the likelihood of strokes. And so on.

In summary: the coronavirus spike protein does its damage by means of inducing endothelial dysfunction. It should come as no surprise that recognized risk factors for severe COVID-19—age, hypertension, obesity, diabetes, chronic lung disease, chronic heart disease, and heart failure—involve endothelial dysfunction as well.

The vast majority of cases of COVID-19 resolve themselves without any lasting ill effects. But for the unlucky few who develop the severe form of the disease, this virus is indeed a formidable enemy.

How the Vax Works

Histories of vaccination usually start with Edward Jenner, the English country doctor who discovered that insertion of infectious matter from cowpox pustules (or *variolae vaccinae,* in Latin) provides protection against smallpox. In 1796 Dr. Jenner tested this technique on an eight-year-old boy, James Phipps, and after twenty subsequent inoculations with smallpox the lad remained disease-free.

Now at this point, the reader could be forgiven for wondering why Dr. Jenner, if he believed so much in his procedure, did not try it out first on himself. That's a fair question, but it remains a fact that Jenner could have become the richest man in the world had he patented his discovery. He chose not to. He just wanted to help people.

In 1798 Dr. Jenner described his work in his treatise *An Inquiry into the Causes and Effects of the Variole Vaccinae, or Cow-Pox,*[69] and the rest, as they say, is history. Jenner's gift to the world led to the complete elimination of the most terrible disease ever to afflict mankind.

The term "vaccination" was introduced by Dr. Jenner's friend Richard Dunn in 1800.[70] Eighty years later, pioneer germ fighter Louis Pasteur called his concoction of attenuated cholera bacteria a "vaccine,"[71] and the definition of a vaccine as a preparation of attenuated or dead pathogens became the generally accepted meaning of the word—at least until very recently.

The Pfizer and Moderna shots would not have qualified as "vaccines" under this definition. These preparations contain no pathogens, dead or alive, nor even parts of pathogens. Rather, they consist of the mRNA sequence for the spike protein, synthesized in a cell-free system and enclosed within a capsule of lipid nanoparticles, which enable it to be taken up by living cells. Because mRNA is an unstable molecule, manufactured just in time to meet the ever-changing needs of the cell, mRNA vaccines must be stored at ultracold temperatures. Moderna states that its product should be stored at minus twenty Celsius, while Pfizer recommends an even chillier minus eighty.

This technology was made possible by two key discoveries. In the late 1980's, Robert Malone, a researcher at the Salk Institute for Biological Studies, developed a new type of lipid capsule for transfecting cells with foreign RNA, and he was the first to suggest that RNA might one day serve as a drug.[72] In the early 1990's, University of Pennsylvania biochemist Katalin Karikó found that modifying the chemical structure of the nucleoside bases that make up mRNA protects them from attack from the body's immune system. This eliminated two potential problems with mRNA therapeutics—degradation of mRNA by the body's own enzymes, and harm resulting from an overstimulated immune response.

After injection into the body, the mRNA forces the cells to produce the spike protein, in the hopes that this protein will stimulate white blood cells called B-cells (so-called because they mature in the bone marrow) to make antibodies—protein molecules which bind to the viral proteins and inactivate the virus and/or target it for destruction by other white blood cells. As world-famous medical expert Bill Gates helpfully explained in an essay in the *Washington Post*, "An RNA vaccine essentially turns your body into its own vaccine manufacturing unit."[73]

The molecule the antibody binds to is called the antigen. Your body can make literally trillions of different types of antibodies, each specific for a specific type of antigen. Your body can make antibodies to substances not even found in nature. And yet you have only about twenty thousand different genes in your genome. (That's all the genes you have, not just the ones for antibodies.)

How is this possible? The short answer is your genome codes not for entire antibodies but for parts of antibodies, which then are shuffled around to make this dizzying variety of combinations possible.

So when a virus or any other types of pathogen invades your body, you likely already will have antibodies on the shelf that can bind to this invader. A process known as fine-tuning increases the closeness of fit between the antibody and the antigen. The genes for antibody proteins are especially prone to mutation. Some of these mutations, just by chance, will tighten the attachment between antibody and antigen. The closer the fit between antibody and antigen, the faster the cell producing that antibody will divide, increasing the chance for more mutations producing an even closer fit, and so on and so forth in a positive feedback process.

Then, after the infection is conquered, especially long-lived cells called memory B-cells remain for years and even decades, serving as a reservoir for antibodies already fine-tuned to that particular invader. That is why once you have recovered from an infection by a given pathogen, your body may well conquer any re-infection by that same pathogen before you even have a chance to develop symptoms.

Getting back to the spike protein: this molecule consists of a chain of exactly 1,237 different amino acid residues strung together in a specific sequence. In both the Pfizer and the Moderna shots, the mRNA sequence that codes for the spike protein has been altered slightly, by substituting two proline residues for the amino acid residues normally present in positions 986 and 987. This is done in order to stabilize the protein in its prefusion conformation, ensuring that the antibodies produced bind to the spike protein before it has a chance to bind to ACE2 and begin the process of destruction inflicted on the body.

Some of the nucleoside bases in the mRNA sequence have been altered chemically as well. We have already seen that mRNA molecules are ephemeral, and are quickly degraded by enzymes which are ubiquitous in living organisms. The modification of the nucleoside bases prolongs the life of the mRNA, and dampens the body's normal response to foreign RNA's, which might lead to dangerous overstimulation of the immune system.

What are the purported advantages of mRNA "vaccines" over conventional vaccines? Well, for one thing, these products are manufactured in a cell-free system, from off-the-shelf chemicals, obviating the time-consuming (and potentially dangerous) process of culturing and working with pathogenic organisms. This enables a lot of product to be brought to market in a short period of time. The injections cause the body to produce the spike protein only, reducing the possibility of the body producing antibodies that bind to other viral proteins without disabling the virus, hopefully reducing the possibility of antibody-dependent enhancement (vide infra). The mRNA is believed to disappear quickly from the body, as is the spike protein, and as the spike protein becomes more scarce, this is expected to lead to the development of high-affinity antibodies. Subsequent booster shots are then expected to increase the levels of these high-affinity antibodies.

Finally, and perhaps the most important reason of all: Once this type of platform is created, it could be easily modified to force the body to produce just about any kind of protein. As Moderna boasted on its website:

> Recognizing the broad potential of RNA science, we set out to create an mRNA technology platform that functions very much like an operating system on a computer. It is designed so it can plug and play interchangeably with different programs. In our case, the "program" or "app" is our mRNA drug—the unique mRNA sequence that codes for a protein.
>
> When we have a concept for a new mRNA medicine and begin research, fundamental components are already in place.

Generally, the only thing that changes from one potential mRNA medicine to another is the coding region—the actual genetic code that instructs ribosomes to make protein. Utilizing these instruction sets gives our investigational mRNA medicines a software-like quality.[74]

I downloaded this page on 3 April 2022. When I checked the Moderna website again on 24 May, all the talk about "software" and "apps" had been deleted, to be replaced with much more anodyne language.

But never mind that for now. It is indisputable that the mRNA platform has the potential to be quickly modified to produce any number of different proteins. Now at this point, the reader could be forgiven for wondering if we may now expect to be plied with hundreds of different "vaccines" hastily rushed to market in a matter of months, but again, never mind that for now.

The question is this: Could there be a downside to hijacking people's cellular machinery to churn out unknown quantities of the toxic spike protein? And how would we know if there was?

How the Vax May Kill

The CDC maintains a database called the Vaccine Adverse Event Reporting System, or VAERS. There are two recognized limitations to post-market reporting systems such as this. On the one hand, these systems are generally believed to capture only between one and ten percent of adverse events. On the other hand, anyone can report an event to VAERS (although intentionally filing a false report is a criminal offense). So these reports are not considered proof of causality. Nevertheless, there are recognized ways of extracting a signal from the raw data.

Proportional Report Ratio (PRR) analysis is a method by which the number of adverse events of a specific type (e.g., myocarditis) associated with a given drug is divided by the total number of adverse events associated with that drug. This ratio is then compared to that of the comparator drugs (in the case of the covid vax, the comparator would be all non-covid vaccines). If the PRR of a given drug is twice that of the comparator, this is considered a signal meriting further investigation.

Given what we already know about the spike protein, we might expect signal detection analysis to reveal the vax rollout was accompanied by a rise in adverse events affecting the lungs, the circulatory system, the nervous system, the kidneys, and the liver. But the potential for damage doesn't stop there.

We already noted that the enzyme ACE produces the hormone Angiotensin II, which promotes cell proliferation, fibrosis, angiogenesis, and cell migration. Cell proliferation and fibrosis lead to the formation of tumors. Angiogenesis provides the blood supply to feed those tumors. Cell migration enables tumor cells move around the body—a process known as metastasis, the process by which tumors become cancers.

ACE2, by contrast, opposes the action of ACE and inhibits cell proliferation, fibrosis, angiogenesis, and cell migration, and is a known inhibitor of cancer cell growth in lung cancer, breast cancer, colon cancer, and pancreatic cancer. A low level of ACE2 expression is a known indicator of poor prognosis in cases of hepatocellular carcinoma. We might expect the vax rollout to be accompanied by a rise in reported cases of cancer.

The spike protein may ravage by other means as well. A paper in *Immunologic Research* published online in September 2020 examined the amino acid sequence of the spike protein and found hundreds of hexapeptide sequences (six amino acids strung together) and dozens of heptapeptide sequences (seven amino acids long) shared between the spike protein and human proteins. The same level of shared resemblance was found between the spike protein and the mouse proteome. However, this level of similarity was much lower for animals (rats, rabbits, cats, dogs, moneys, apes) on which SARS-2-CoV has little or no effect.[75] These were surprising findings indeed, given that we obviously are much closer related to monkeys and apes than we are to mice.

The conclusion was inescapable: natural selection has altered the genetic instructions of the viral protein to make it resemble those of our own, enabling the virus to blend in and escape detection by the human immune system—a process known as "molecular mimicry."[76]

You may well ask, So what? Well, scientists had long believed that our immune system weeds out B-cells that produce antibodies which recognize the self. Now they know this isn't always true. Your blood does contain B-cells which can initiate an immune response against the self, but the activity of these cells normally is held in check—no one really knows how.

But what happens when these cells encounter the spike protein which contains amino acid sequences they have been programmed to recognize and attack? Can they become activated and attack not just the viral protein but your own cells as well? That seems like a reasonable conjecture. We might expect the vax rollout to be accompanied by a rise in inflammatory and autoimmune disease.

So what happened after the covid vaccines were rushed to the market and hundreds of millions of human bodies were turned into factories for manufacturing the toxic spike protein? That's a good question.

In January of 2021, the CDC promised to carry out Proportional Report Ratio analysis of VAERS data weekly. But they did not make the data available to the public until January of 2023—and when they did, the results were eye-opening, to say the least. Details to follow.

Original Antigenic Sin and Antibody-Dependent Enhancement

There are other ways the vax may have potential to cause harm. Thomas Francis Jr., the scientist who first isolated the influenza virus, noted that when subjects are exposed to a particular strain of flu virus, the antibodies they express bind most strongly not to that particular strain but rather to the strain that was most prevalent when the subject was a child. It was as if once the immune system is trained to "see" a particular strain of virus, it can "see" only that strain and no other. Dr. Thomas coined the phrase "original antigenic sin" (OAS) to describe this process.

Since then, original antigenic sin has been documented for a variety of viral infections, not just in humans but in other animals as well. How this process happens no one really knows, but one possible explanation is this: when a new strain of a virus the body has already encountered invades the body, the antibodies from the memory B-cells bind to the new strain—albeit weakly. These memory B-cells become activated and divide, creating more B-cells which continue to produce antibodies which bind weakly to the new strain, while other B-cells that might have done a better job never get the chance to do so. This could lead to a sub-optimal immune response or, even worse, to another problem called antibody-dependent enhancement (ADE). This is when the immune response goes awry and actually makes the body more vulnerable to an invader.

Antibody-dependent enhancement happens when the B-cells produce antibodies which bind to a viral protein only weakly, or bind to the wrong part of a protein and fail to neutralize the virus. The antibody-antigen complex then binds to a special type of receptor on the white blood cell and is engulfed by that cell. The covering of non-neutralizing antibodies has been likened to a Trojan horse, allowing the virus to enter the cell undetected and hijack that cell's machinery of replication, transcription, and translation to make more virions, resulting in a more severe infection that would have occurred had the body never been exposed to the viral protein in the first place.

Antibody-dependent enhancement of viral infections has been documented in kittens, ferrets, mice, monkeys, and humans. This process occurs primarily in positive-strand RNA viruses—including SARS-CoV-1, which is closely related to the virus causing the current pandemic—along with the viruses causing Zika, yellow fever, Dengue fever, Respiratory Syncytial Virus (RSV) infection, and AIDS.

The vax was rushed on to the market without anything like adequate follow-up to investigate these possibilities.

Were We Warned?

In a word: Yes.

In July of 2020, a team of Harvard researchers wrote in the journal *Nature Biotechnology*:

> Whether SARS-CoV-2 can cause ADE is an open question. ADE in individuals with multiple SARS-CoV-2 infections or cross-reactivity to common-cold-causing CoV's will likely take several years. However, given that ADE has been observed with the closely-related SARS-CoV, we believe that the question of ADE effects in SARS-CoV-2 should be urgently resolved using experimental immunology.[77]

The next month a team of Stanford researchers wrote in *Nature*:

> At present, there are no known clinical findings, immunological assays, or biomarkers that can differentiate any severe viral infection from immune-enhanced disease.
>
> Because ADE of disease cannot be reliably predicted after either vaccination or treatment with antibodies—regardless of what virus is the causative agent—it will be essential to depend on careful analysis of safety in humans as immune interventions for COVID-19 move forward.[78]

Two days before the FDA advisory panel voted to authorize the Pfizer shot for emergency use, Patrick Whelan, Associate Professor of Clinical Pediatrics at the University of California Los Angeles, wrote to the panel:

> It appears that the viral spike protein that is the target of the major SARS-CoV-2 vaccines is also one of the key agents

causing the damage to distant organs that may include the brain, heart, lung, and kidney. Before any of these vaccines are approved for widespread use in humans, it is important to assess in vaccinated subjects the effects of vaccination on the heart.

As important as it is to quickly arrest the spread of the virus by immunizing the population, it would be vastly worse if hundreds of millions of people were to suffer long-lasting or even permanent damage to their brain or heart micro-vasculature as a result of failing to appreciate in the short-term an unintended effect of full-length spike protein-based vaccines on these other organs.[79]

Early in the vax rollout, two researchers from the University of Texas Health Science Center issued these words of caution:

OAS is the double-edged sword of memory; it can provide an avenue to protection against a novel strain of a pathogen or create an obstacle to the elicitation of protective immunity. What this means for COVID-19 is yet to be fully deter-mined, but this important consequence of the immense powers of immunological memory and specificity must be considered when assessing population-level immunity and vaccine efficacy.[80]

Yet again, all of these words of caution fell upon deaf ears.

* * *

In summary: there is every reason to believe most of the pernicious effects of the coronavirus infection can also be caused by the vax. In addition, the mRNA products may have the potential actually to diminish the body's immune response to the coronavirus, by means of either original antigenic sin or antibody-dependent enhancement, or both. And yet, we are assured the Pfizer and Moderna shots are safe and effective, based on evidence manufactured and controlled by the same companies that manufacture these products.

What do we know about these companies, and do they deserve the blind trust we are being demanded to place in them?

SARS-CoV-2 (RAAS)

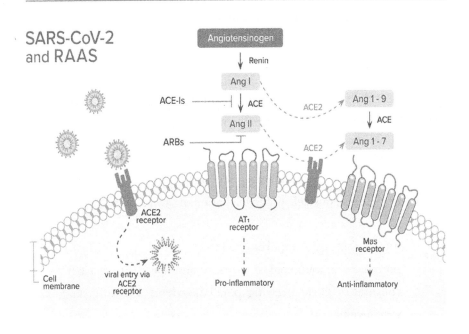

The association between SARS-CoV-2 and
the Renin-Angiotensin-Aldosterone System (RAAS)[81]

CHAPTER THREE

Hope Changes Lives

We Do the Right Thing

Imagine (God forbid) the worst thing that can happen to anyone has happened to you. Your son is having difficulty adjusting to his new school. You take him to your trusted family doctor, who prescribes medication for him. Less than week later he goes into his room and hangs himself from a coat hook barely higher than he is tall.

Now imagine you go to court to try to obtain a modicum of justice for your boy—and the next thing you know, forensic experts hired by the corporation that manufactured the drug he had been taking are coming into your home to look for semen samples on the carpet—because, obviously, your son's death had nothing to do with the pills he had been taking but rather was a case of "auto-erotic asphyxiation."

This nightmare scenario actually happened. The boy in question was thirteen-year-old Matthew Miller, and the drug in question was Zoloft, manufactured by pharmaceutical industry giant Pfizer.

Zoloft is marketed by Pfizer as an "antidepressant" and is classified as a Selective Serotonin Reuptake Inhibitor (SSRI)—a member of the same class of drugs to which Prozac and Paxil belong. Zoloft was approved by the FDA for treatment of major depressive disorder in 1991. FDA rules stipulate that before a drug can be approved, the manufacturer must submit two clinical trials demonstrating it performs significantly better than placebo. That may sound pretty good until you realize there can be any number of negative trials, which just don't count. In the case of Zoloft, six trials had to be performed to get the requisite two positive ones.[82]

Pfizer later sponsored two trials on the effects of Zoloft on children. Both yielded negative results. These two trials were combined to get one positive one which was published in *JAMA* in 2003.[83] Pfizer's own data showed a tripling of behavioral problems, including aggression and suicidality, in children given the active drug.

Today Zoloft and all SSRI antidepressants carry a black-box warning of increased risk of suicidal thoughts and behaviors in children and young adults up the age of twenty-five years. The reason this effect is supposed to magically turn itself off after the twenty-fifth birthday has never been explained.

This black-box warning was not available at the time Matt met his demise. Matt's doctor had been working as a paid speaker for Pfizer—a fact his parents were unaware of until it came out in the course of the trial.

Dr. Healy testified as an expert witness for the plaintiffs at the trial. I asked Dr. Healy, Was Matt Miller's death something Pfizer could reasonably have been expected to foresee? Here is what he had to say:

> They had very clear evidence, and there were internal documents that made it clear that they knew that from ten years before the drug came on the market. It was clear that they knew their drug could cause people to commit suicide.
>
> When they gave the drug to healthy volunteers, some of them became suicidal, and Pfizer reviewed these trials and said, It's very clear that our drug has caused this in this case. And it's also well known that drugs like ours can cause agitation and can cause people to become suicidal.

Pfizer knew.

This sad sordid story is hardly the only example of Pfizer putting profits ahead of people.

Pfizer was founded in New York City in 1849 by two German immigrants: Charles Pfizer and his cousin Charles Erhart. Their first product was santonin, an anthelmintic compound. Since then the venture has grown into a corporation spanning the globe with some fifty billion dollars in annual revenues.

The company's website greets visitors with the slogan "Hope changes lives." Elsewhere, we are informed, "At Pfizer, we do the right thing because patients' lives depend on us." But Pfizer's track record tells another story.

On 2 September 2009, the United States Department of Justice announced that Pfizer had agreed to pay $2.3 billion to settle claims of illegal marketing of four of its drugs: the analgesic Bextra, the antipsychotic drug Geodon, the antibiotic Zyvox, and the anticonvulsant Lyrica.[84] This was the largest such settlement in history, although it has since been eclipsed by the $3 billion settlement paid by fellow industry giant GlaxoSmithKline three years later.

Most of the allegations centered on Pfizer's blockbuster drug Bextra. This nostrum was originally developed by G.D. Searle, a subsidiary of Monsanto. In 2000 Monsanto merged with Pharmacia & Upjohn to form Pharmacia Corporation. In 2001, the FDA approved Bextra, but only for three indications: osteoarthritis, rheumatoid arthritis, and menstrual cramps.[85] The FDA specifically declined to approve the drug for post-surgical pain, but for some reason they never told the public that their own secret documents had shown the drug caused "an excess of serious adverse events, including death."[86]

Undaunted, the company enlisted the services of Scirex, a clinical research organization owned by the advertising firm Omnicom, which commissioned a study which found Bextra was superior to Percocet for pain experienced after wisdom tooth extraction. The study was published in the May 2002 issue of the *Journal of the American Dental Association.*

Eric Topol, then Chairman of the Cleveland Clinic Department of Cardiovascular Medicine, noted that the study compared a single dose of Bextra to a single dose of Percocet, ignoring the fact that doctors have always known the effects of Percocet wear off after four to six hours. He called it a "contrived comparison," noting he found it "quite disquieting" that Scirex was owned by an advertising agency, and added "If this is where clinical research is headed, that would be a terrible negative trajectory."[87]

Two months after the study was published, Pharmacia was bought out by Pfizer. The latter's commitment to "doing the right thing" was demonstrated when Pfizer decided to renege on a deal negotiated two years previously by Pharmacia, which had promised to license patents for its AIDS drug Rescriptor to the Concept Foundation, a not-for-profit organization which distributes essential medicines to poor countries. Pfizer claimed that there were better drugs available for the treatment of AIDS, and that the decision to deep-six the agreement had been mutual.[88]

This news came as a surprise to Joachim Oehler, Chief Executive of the Concept Foundation. "This is hypocrisy," he said of Pfizer's decision.[89]

Joseph Gonzi, a consultant on AIDS medicines for the International Dispensary Association which had helped negotiate the deal, concurred. "I would have taken [Rescriptor], if they had given it to me," he told a reporter. Meanwhile Pfizer continued to sell the drug in the United States and Canada along with other countries. US sales receipts for the drug in 2002 totaled $7.4 million.[90]

Meanwhile, the corporate skullduggery surrounding Bextra by no means came to an end after Pfizer acquired Pharmacia. Pfizer illegally promoted the off-label prescribing of the drug, exhorting its sales reps to tell doctors that the FDA had given the drug "a clean bill of health"[91] and wooing prescribers with all-expenses paid "meetings" at luxury resorts in the Caribbean where they listened to presentations where paid shills touted the drug, in between rounds of massages, golfing, and other assorted types of fun in the sun. Thousands of docs may have attended these junkets, which included "honoraria" of up to $2,000 apiece.[92]

On 7 April 2005, the FDA ordered Pfizer to pull Bextra from the market, citing concerns over heart problems as well as a dangerous skin condition caused by this drug.[93] On 17 October of that year, Pfizer announced it would pay $894 million to settle lawsuits brought by patients (and their families) who claimed to have been harmed by Bextra and a related drug, Celebrex.[94]

A year and a half later, the DoJ announced the $2.3 billion settlement over claims of illegal marketing, trumpeting in a press release, "Today's enormous fine demonstrates that such blatant and continued disregard of the law will not be tolerated."[95] Officials called the company a "repeat offender," noting that this was the fourth such settlement paid out by the company in the past decade.[96]

Pfizer's legal representatives had already said in court "The company's intent was pure," and was intended merely to foster a legal exchange of scientific information among doctors.[97]

Former FDA Deputy Commissioner Scott Gottlieb complained that government prosecutors were "increasingly criminalizing what reasonable people might argue is a reasonable exchange of important clinical information between drug companies and doctors."[98] Dr. Gottlieb would later go on to become Commissioner of the FDA, a position he held until he stepped down in 2019 to join the board of directors of Pfizer.

Pfizer General Counsel Amy Schulman told the Associated Press the settlement brings "final closure to significant legal matters and helps enhance our focus on what we do best—discovering, developing, and delivering innovative medicines."[99]

But that was not the end of the story. Seven months later, the DoJ accepted a guilty plea for criminal charges related to the illegal marketing of Bextra. But, incredibly, the plea was entered not on behalf of Pfizer, and certainly not on behalf of anyone who had worked for that company.

Rather, the plea was entered by Pharmacia & Upjohn Co. Inc., a subsidiary of a subsidiary of a subsidiary of Pfizer, a shell corporation which existed for no other purpose than to plead guilty to the charges.[100]

As a CNN story put it:

> Imagine being charged with a crime, but an imaginary friend takes the rap for you.
>
> That is essentially what happened when Pfizer, the world's largest pharmaceutical company, was caught illegally marketing Bextra.[101]

Why was this done? Federal law stipulates that companies convicted of major health care fraud are barred from participating in Medicare and Medicaid. Prosecutors noted that this likely would lead to Pfizer's collapse, with cascading effects: disrupting the flow of the company's nostrums to Medicare and Medicaid recipients, causing Pfizer employees to lose their jobs, and creating significant loss for Pfizer shareholders.[102]

In effect, the feds were arguing the corporate behemoth was too big to fail.

Pfizer's chief compliance Officer Doug Lankler told CNN "I can tell you, unequivocally, that Pfizer perceived the Bextra matter as an incredibly serious one."[103]

The settlement amounted to about three weeks' worth of sales receipts for Pfizer.

Two years later, we got to find out just how seriously Pfizer takes these matters when John MacArthur, publisher of *Harper's*, revealed that the company had pulled "between $400,000 and a million dollars" worth of advertising from the magazine after they ran a piece that was perceived as unflattering to Pfizer's blockbuster drug Zoloft.[104]

Of course, that's just good business sense. But it does raise questions about whether we can indeed trust Pfizer to "change patients' lives," at least for the better. It also raises questions about why direct-to-consumer advertising of prescription drugs is even allowed in this country, and whether we can trust the pronouncements of the legacy media addicted to drug company largesse in a time of falling ad revenues.

But all of this pales when compared to the mendacity the company displayed in the marketing of its blockbuster stop-smoking drug Chantix.

Rages That Make No Sense at All

- In September of 2007, thirty-four-year-old musician Carter Albrecht became inexplicably agitated and violent, screaming and kicking at the door of a neighbor's home. The neighbor responded by firing a shot through the door, and Carter died at the scene. Police declined to file any charges in the case.[105]

- In May of 2009, thirty-four-year-old Sean Wain of Economy, Pennsylvania, murdered his wife of fourteen years with a shotgun blast before turning the gun on himself, leaving their four small children orphaned. Neighbors and the family pastor said they had seen no sign of any marital discord prior to the shootings.[106]

- In July of 2010, thirty-three-year-old delivery driver Andrew Case of Fordingbridge, England, stabbed his wife Vicki to death, then smothered their two little girls and covered all three victims with a blanket before hanging himself.[107]

- In December of that same year, forty-nine-year-old Darwin Stout of Eugene, Oregon, stabbed his only son to death, then used the knife to end his own life. Two days earlier, Stout had entered a mental hospital for evaluation but was discharged after a nurse practitioner and a social worker interviewed him and concluded he was not a danger to himself or others.[108]

Each one of these tragedies took place shortly after the killer began taking Pfizer's blockbuster stop-smoking drug Chantix.

In its first full year on the market, Chantix racked up an impressive $883 million in sales.[109] Advertisements for Chantix chirped "Quitting can be different this time." And how.

Chantix was approved by the FDA on 11 May 2006, even though Pfizer's own studies which formed the basis for the approval of the drug—in which they did everything they could to tilt the balance in favor of their product and against placebo—showed the company's nostrum was of no help to the great majority of patients who took it. A story in CBS News quoted one expert as saying the drug would prove to be most valuable for smokers who had tried Zyban or nicotine replacement therapy but failed to quit[110]—ignoring the fact that Pfizer had excluded such patients from its trials.

A study published by Thomas Moore and his colleagues at the non-profit Institute for Safe Medication Practices found that by the fourth quarter of 2007, Chantix surpassed all other drugs for serious events reported to the FDA, including but not limited to hostility, aggression, paranoia, hallucinations, psychosis, heart arrhythmias, heart attacks, visual disturbances, seizures, falls, traffic accidents, homicidal ideation, suicidal ideation, and suicide attempts, along with twenty-eight actual suicides.[111]

The Institute notified the FDA,[112] which in July of 2009 issued an alert and required Pfizer to include a black box warning—the strongest sanction possible short of banning a drug—on all packages of Chantix, cautioning users and health professionals to be on the lookout for changes in behavior, hostility, agitation, depressed mood, suicidal thoughts and behavior, and attempted suicide.[113]

In May of 2010, Moore and his colleagues at the ISMP released another report providing further evidence for the link between Chantix and violence.[114] They examined case reports of violent thoughts or actions towards others, and from these extracted twenty-six cases that qualified for a diagnosis of substance intoxication. The twenty-six case reports included three completed suicides. In every case, the acts or thoughts of violence towards others appeared to be both unprovoked and inexplicable. Most of the perpetrators had no previous history of violence, and most of them were middle-aged women—not a group known for its propensity towards violent behavior. Furthermore, the intended or actual victims were anyone who happened to be nearby—a daughter, a boyfriend, a fiancé, a husband, neighbors, co-workers, even a policeman.

The paper provides details of the bizarre and random nature of some of these acts of violence. A matron struck her seventeen-year-old daughter in the mouth while her daughter was driving a car; the woman's young granddaughter was also present. A forty-two-year-old man punched a stranger in the mouth at a bowling alley; the stranger and his two friends responded by knocking the man's teeth out. A young woman started beating her boyfriend as he lay sleeping beside her because "he looked so peaceful," she later tried to kill herself.

Moore and his colleagues explained that the increased risk of violence associated with Chantix could not be due solely to the effects of nicotine withdrawal, noting that many of violence case reports originated during the first week of treatment, before the smoking quit date.

What's more, fourteen of these case reports provided dechallenge information; in thirteen of these, symptoms resolved a few days after Chantix was discontinued, while in the fourteenth, symptoms had improved but not fully resolved at the time of the report. In three of these cases, rechallenge information was provided as well; in all three cases symptoms reappeared when the drug was re-started. This is considered proof of a cause-and-effect relationship.

The same month the challenge-dechallenge rechallenge case histories were published, the FDA sent a letter of warning to Pfizer, accusing them of a whole slew of irregularities in the company's reporting of adverse drug experiences with respect to a wide variety of drugs. These include failure to submit adverse drug experience reports to the FDA as required, misclassifying and/or downgrading reports to non-serious without reasonable justification, and inadequate written procedures for the surveillance, receipt, and reporting of adverse events. The letter went on for six pages, detailing a pattern of alleged violations, many of which, the FDA claimed, had already been brought to Pfizer's attention before.

In December of that year, another report by the ISMP provided further evidence of a link between Chantix and violence.[115] Moore and his colleagues analyzed adverse drug event reports submitted to the FDA for the period beginning in 2004 and ending with the third quarter of 2009. Only drugs for which at least two hundred adverse events were reported were included in their analysis—a total of 484 drugs in all. For each of these drugs, Moore et al. tabulated the incidence of violence case reports, which they defined as violence-related symptoms, physical abuse, physical assault, homicidal ideation, and homicide.

For the majority of these 484 drugs, there were no violence case reports. For most of the rest, there were only one or two such reports. Chantix stood out from the pack with a whopping 408 violence case reports, or twenty-one percent of the total. The proportion of violence case reports for Chantix was eighteen times the average for all other drugs.

The following May, yet another report by the ISMP noted a spike in the number of violence case reports for the third quarter of 2010 due to a large number of adverse events which occurred in previous quarters but had not been previously tabulated by the FDA due to irregularities in Pfizer's reporting system.[116]

How did this happen? The FDA's expedited review system requires drug companies to report within fifteen days adverse events that are both serious and unexpected. Less-serious and expected events are submitted quarterly, in so-called "periodic reports." Pfizer was including suicides in the periodic reports. Moreover, Pfizer was lumping individual reports along with case summaries into a single text file, and these individual reports were not tabulated by the FDA.

These adverse events included 150 suicides, more than doubling the total number of suicides linked to Chantix.

All this raises a question: Is suicide of Chantix users an "expected event?"

In February of 2013, Pfizer announced it was paying out $273 million to settle eighty percent of the 2,700 state and federal lawsuits filed on behalf of people claiming to have been harmed by Chantix. In an SEC filing, company officials estimated that settling the remaining cases would cost another $15 million dollars.[117]

In September of 2014 Thomas Moore and his colleagues at the ISMP issued still another report analyzing adverse event reports from 2007 through the third quarter of 2013. Chantix accounted for more cases of suicidal ideation, self-harm, and homicidal ideation than any other drug, by a more than three-fold margin. For cases of homicidal ideation, the difference was a whopping five-fold.[118]

On October 16, 2014, the FDA convened a hearing to consider whether or not to drop the black-box warning from Chantix. Christopher Wohlberg, Vice President and Safety Surveillance & Risk Management Group Head for Pfizer, presented the results of eighteen randomized clinical trials (all funded by Pfizer) and four observational studies. "The current control data show no evidence of increased risk of serious neuropsychiatric events when compared to placebo, bupropion, or NRT," Dr. Wohlberg testified, concluding it was "time to unring the alarm bell" on Chantix.[119]

Dr. Wohlberg's testimony ignored the fact that the Pfizer trial data was not available for inspection, so we just have to take their word for all this, and also ignored the fact that tens of millions of people have successfully quit smoking without any chemical assistance whatsoever—a point that would seem to undercut the urgency of Wohlberg's demand.

Dr. Wohlberg was followed by Thomas Moore of the Institute for Safe Medication Practices, who began by highlighting the human cost behind some relatively innocuous-sounding labels like "sleep disturbances," stating, "Some of them are the most horrifying dreams that people can actually not speak about."

He then blasted the industry experts whose testimony preceded his:

> Now I was here this morning and wondered—I was listening to some of this—to be frank, whether I was in Alice in Wonderland. So we have a manufacturer who, let's face the facts, paid 2,500 Chantix victims of neuropsychiatric side effects rather than try a single case in court. And now we hear a scientific presentation that ignores most of the evidence that says it doesn't cause psychiatric side effects.
>
> In 10 or 15 years of doing this kind of work, we just have not seen anything like this kind of drug.

Kim Witczak also testified at the Chantix hearings, noting that not one of the 2,700 plaintiffs who had accepted the settlement was there to testify, nor were their lawyers. She quoted from one plaintiff who settled: "I sincerely wish I could tell my story publicly, but like the other 2,700 people who accepted Pfizer's settlement, I am bound from saying anything." Witczak went on to lament that the Chantix settlement meant that "22 million pages of documents and dozens of key dispositions may be forever lost without some sort of intervention."

In the end, the FDA panel voted eleven-to-seven to keep the black-box warning on Chantix,[120] and in March of 2015 issued another warning, stating that Chantix can decrease tolerance to alcohol, leading to increased drunkenness, unusual or aggressive behavior, and blackouts, and that rare cases of seizures had been recorded in users who either had no previous history of seizures, or whose seizures had been well-controlled.[121]

Kim later told me:

> This is part of my big message to attorneys: if you don't figure out a way to get the evidence released from under seal, it will

forever stay under seal and all the public health knowledge is lost and the problem persists.

In a telephone interview, Moore summed up matters thusly:

> I think our society and our legal system are not ready to think about and understand that drugs are capable of making people suicidal and violent. This drug as well as other drugs can cause people to think about homicide, to explode into rages that make no sense at all.

On 16 September 2016, the FDA voted to remove the black-box warning,[122] and Chantix remains on the market. For the year 2019, the last full year the drug remained on patent, it netted Pfizer over one billion dollars in sales.[123]

Changing the World of Medicine

Moderna's website boasts "We are changing the world of medicine," adding:

> Our mRNA platform, with its speed, scale, and flexibility, is uniquely suited to tackle current and emerging pathogens that threaten global health.

Moderna is a portmanteau of the words "Modified" and "RNA." This company was formed as the result of a collaborative effort by two men: Derrick Rossi, Assistant Professor of Biochemistry at Harvard Medical School, and Noubar Afeyan, CEO of the venture capital firm Flagship Ventures. Dr. Rossi had used Robert Malone's technique of mRNA transfection to convert cells taken from the body into stem cells, which are capable of differentiating into any of the other cell types in the body. He presented his findings to Afeyan, who wasn't interested in stem cell research but who saw other potential uses for this technology—and so

Moderna was born, with a $40 million stake from Flagship. The following year, Stéphane Bancel, CEO of the French biotechnology firm BioMérieux, was lured away from his position to helm the new startup.

In his book *A Shot to Save the World*, author Gregory Zuckerman repeats a claim by Moderna co-founder Rossi, who says Bancel asked him to disclose some of the research he was doing for Boston Children's Hospital so Moderna could file patents on the work. Zuckerman quotes Rossi as follows:

> The work is their property. He was asking me to steal from a
> hospital that treats children.
> Stéphane is someone without a moral compass.[124]

Bancel and Dr. Rossi locked horns repeatedly until, like many an entrepreneur, Rossi learned the hard way that those who found corporations are not the ones who get to run them. Eventually he faded into the background, directing most of his attention to other ventures, while Bancel emerged the undisputed King of the Hill, with free rein to continue expanding his empire.

In March of 2013, drug company goliath AstraZeneca forked over $240 million to Moderna for exclusive rights for five years for dozens of different drugs, none of which even yet existed.[125] Other investors lined up in hopes of cashing in, and by 2016, the company was valued at $4.5 billion—without a single product ever even having made it to Phase I trials.[126] Bancel acquired a reputation as a hard taskmaster, with former employees complaining about a pressure-cooker atmosphere and arbitrary firings, but perhaps this is to be expected from a company that aspires to be on the cutting edge of science.

"Moderna's strategy is to aggressively commercialize its mRNA platform for patients in need," Bancel told reporters.[127] However, as is often the case in life, the devil turned out to be in the details. The sweet spot between too little and too much of a dose of mRNA proved to be elusive.

Too little provides no therapeutic effect, while too much ramps the body's immune response to dangerous levels. On 10 January 2017, *STAT* reported that one of Moderna's most promising products (a treatment for a one-in-a-million inborn error of metabolism called Crigler-Najjer Syndrome) had been placed on the back burner indefinitely.[128]

Bancel was undeterred. "mRNA is like software," he told *STAT*. "You can just turn the crank and get a lot of products going into development."[129] The company turned its efforts to vaccines.

This move came as a surprise to some observers—vaccines have long been seen as a loss leader in the pharmaceutical market—but it left Moderna in an enviable position after a new form of pneumonia was reported by doctors on the other side of the world in December of 2019. By mid-2021, the company was valued at a staggering one hundred billion dollars.[130] Total revenues for that year exceeded $18.5 billion[131]—not bad for an outfit with only one product. The picture was even brighter for 2022, with the firm raking in a cool $6.1 billion for the first quarter.[132]

Spikevax remains Moderna's only product to have reached the market, although the company has forty-four others in various stages of development—all of them mRNA vaccines.

Translating Science into Survival

BioNTech is a contraction of Biopharmaceutical New Technologies. Their website informs visitors "We are translating science into survival by developing new immunotherapies."

The company was founded in Mainz, Germany, 2008, by the husband-and-wife team of researchers Uğur Şahin and Özlem Türeci, who wanted to adapt the new technology of modified RNA to produce vaccines for use as individualized cancer therapies. Katalin Karikó, whose work on modified RNA at the University of Pennsylvania had helped make all this possible, joined the firm as Senior Vice President in 2013.

The company scored a major coup in late 2015 when they signed a $1.5 billion contract with French pharmaceutical titan Sanofi for the rights to five discovery-stage cancer immunotherapies.[133] Less than a year later, BioNTech reached a similar accord with Genentech, a subsidiary of the drugmaker Roche, worth another $310 million.[134] Two years after that, the startup entered into yet another agreement, this one with Pfizer, for the development of flu vaccines, to the tune of $400 million.[135]

At this time, after ten years of operation, BioNTech had not brought a single product to the market. But, like Moderna, the company was excellently poised when the new malady from China swept across the globe. For the year 2021, they reported €19 billion in revenues,[136] with a market capitalization worth $62 billion.[137]

To date, Comirnaty remains their only product, although they claim to have another thirty or more products in various stages of development, including ten mRNA vaccines for infectious diseases along mRNA therapeutics for cancer as well as cell therapies, antibodies, and small molecule immunotherapies.[138]

* * *

In summary: the evidence purporting to show the covid shots are safe and effective is manufactured and controlled by three companies, one of which has a long record of hiding data along with an arrant disregard for the law and for human life, and which the United States Department of Justice apparently has deemed too big to fail. The other two had no products on the market prior to 2020, and now have a single product each, with billions and billions of dollars riding on the success or failure of that product. Perhaps a bit of caution is in order here.

CHAPTER FOUR

Staying Silent Is Not the Responsible Option

February–October 2021

The Start is the Start

On Wednesday 3 February, a re-analysis funded by Public Health England (PHE) of data from Israel (a nation noted for the speed and breadth of its vaccine coverage) reported that that the risk of infection actually *increased* in the first nine days after administration of the Pfizer shot, and did not return to baseline level until twenty-one days.[139] There had already been anecdotal evidence this may be the case, in the form of a rash of covid outbreaks and deaths in nursing homes in the UK immediately after vaccination,[140] but now there was confirmation of this by means of hard data.

These disturbing findings become even more disturbing when you realize that the Pfizer and Moderna protocols stipulate that the primary endpoint is covid infection of any severity occurring at least twenty-eight days after the first shot (in the case of the Pfizer vax) or forty-two days (in the case of the Moderna product). Cases that occur before that just don't count, although the drugmakers never explained why these cases shouldn't matter to the patient. Neither Pfizer nor Moderna made any effort to conceal this—it was right there in the trial protocols all along—although nobody at the time seems to have picked up on its significance.

If the vax causes the rate of covid infections to increase, how this happens is obviously nowhere near as important as that it happens. But Pfizer's own data from its Phase I/II trial showed their product caused a precipitous drop in the number of lymphocytes, which did not return to normal until six to eight days later.[141] The lymphocytes are the class of white blood cells which includes the B-cells, which we have already talked about; the T-cells, the other one of the twin pillars of the body's acquired immune response; and the natural killer cells, the shock troops which serve as the body's first line of defense in the war against viral invaders. The drop in lymphocyte count was dose-dependent, proving a cause-and-effect relationship. So the proposed increase in covid infections immediately following the shot certainly is pharmacologically plausible.

This is huge. I asked Dr. Doshi to comment on the trial protocols in which covid infections in the first four or six weeks after administration of the first dose don't count toward the primary endpoint. This is what he had to say:

> Another aspect that's at play in these conversations is the question of what is the appropriate endpoint to be looking at? And so, for example, you must be aware that the trials only start counting cases a week in Pfizer's case, two weeks in Moderna's case, after dose two. Well, in my opinion that's a completely biased trial design. We shouldn't start counting when we think the drug should start to work, we start counting after people receive their dose. We should start counting actually at randomization, when things start. The start is the start. You know—who are we being fair to? Are we being fair to the drug, or are we being fair to the patient?

Three days later, a paper in the *BMJ* summarized mounting evidence confirming that the rate of covid infection actually went up in the days following vaccination.[142] A PHE study concluded that the risk of infection in patients over eighty years of age in the UK increased by as much as forty-eight percent in the first nine days following vaccination.[143] A Danish study reported that the risk of infection in nursing home residents rose by forty percent in the first fourteen days after receiving the vax.[144] This trend had also been noted earlier that month in the minutes of the eighty-third meeting of the Scientific Advisory Group for Emergencies (SAGE).[145] (Bizarrely, the names of many of the experts that helped produce that report had been blacked out before the report was finally released.) Indeed, as the reader should recall, Pfizer's own data submitted for Emergency Use Authorization of the shot reported 409 cases of "suspected COVID-19" in the treatment group in the first seven days following either inoculation, as opposed to only 287 among those given placebo.

No consideration at all was given to the possibility that the shot may be *causing* covid infection in these cases. Pfizer attributed the increase in suspected cases to "vaccine reactogenicity"—and remember, Pfizer's own protocol instructed clinicians specifically not to test participants for covid in such cases. SAGE, for its part, attributed the increases in confirmed cases to "behaviour changes" following vaccination.[146] The *BMJ* followed suit, quoting one expert in the "psychology of emerging health risks" as follows:

> The research has shown that immediately after the first jab, people are more likely to be flouting social distancing, meeting people outside their household or bubble—and meeting them indoors.[147]

Not a shred of data was adduced that actually showed an increase in "flouting social distancing" post-vaccination, by eighty-year-old nursing home residents or anyone else.

Aliens in Their Own Country

Meanwhile, the State of Israel became the first of many nations to implement what came to be known as "vaccine passports." In February of that year, that nation rolled out its "green pass" system, which allowed bearers to access gyms, cultural and sporting events, hotels, and swimming pools, in exchange for divulging to strangers what used to be private medical information. Health Minister Yuli Edelstein warned Israelis "Whoever does not get vaccinated will be left behind."[148]

Similar documents were introduced in dozens of nations on six continents, enabling entry to malls, shopping centers, markets, bars, nightclubs, cruises, restaurants, gyms, saunas, entertainment centers, and the like. The United States never instituted a nationwide vaccine passport (and several states passed laws preemptively banning them), although several states and municipalities did require them, including New York City, New Orleans, and Los Angeles.

Some were enthusiastic about the idea. British television presenter Piers Morgan tweeted:

> Love the idea of covid vaccine passports for everywhere: flights, restaurants, clubs, football, gyms, shops, etc.
>
> It's time covid-denying anti-vaxxer loonies had their bullsh*t bluff called & bar themselves from going anywhere responsible citizens go.

The choice to call these documents "passports" was (perhaps unintentionally) telling. A "passport" is a document that allows the citizen to travel in a foreign country. By identifying these documents as "passports," their proponents were in effect turning the citizenry into aliens in their own country.

Vaccinated People Do Not Carry the Virus

On 16 March I appeared as a guest on Peter Breggin's YouTube Channel. Dr. Breggin, widely known as "The Conscience of Psychiatry," has a long and distinguished history of speaking out against the harms caused by psychiatric medications as well as the benefits of a gentle, empathetic, client-centered approach to those problems with living known as "mental illnesses." The stated reason for my being there was to discuss my book about antidepressants, but we spent most of the time talking about society's panicky, scared response to the covid pandemic. Afterwards, in retaliation, YouTube removed all two hundred of Dr. Breggin's videos.

On 30 March, *Business Insider*[149] reported that CDC Director Rochelle Walensky shared the following good news at a White House Press Briefing:

> Our data from the CDC today suggests that vaccinated people do not carry the virus, don't get sick, and that's not just in the clinical trials, but it's also in real-world data.

The eminent doctor also stressed the importance of getting shots into arms as quickly as possible:

> We know that about 10% of the population that gets sick with COVID-19 has long-haul syndrome, has symptoms beyond three weeks, cardiac challenges, depression and mental-health challenges, pulmonary challenges, renal failure, clotting.

Fortunately, help was on the way. The article concluded with these words of reassurance: "Some long-haul COVID-19 patients are now finding getting vaccinated can help them feel better after many months of such lingering issues." No data were cited in support of this assertion.

Nine New Billionaires

On the first day of April, a Pfizer press release trumpeted the latest safety and efficacy data for the vax, "measured seven days through up to six months after the second dose."[150]

Note the wording: "*Up to six months…*" In fact, by the data cut-off date of 13 March, only twelve thousand participants had made it that far in a trial that originally enrolled forty-four thousand subjects and was slated to last for two full years.

The press release also claimed the incidence of "severe COVID-19" was reduced by either 95.3 percent or one hundred percent, depending on which definition of "severe COVID-19" was used. It did not mention that cases of covid occurring within four weeks after the first dose were not included in this endpoint.[151] Based on these results, Pfizer announced its intention to seek full FDA approval for its product.

On the twenty-sixth of that month, the website military.com reported that fourteen cases of myocarditis had been reported in military health patients after receiving either the Pfizer or the Moderna vax. Only one of these patients developed myocarditis after the first shot, while the remaining thirteen developed the condition after the second—suggesting a dose-dependent relationship. Neither Pfizer nor Moderna responded to requests for comment.[152]

On 4 May, an article in *Science Blogs* attempted to allay people's unfounded fears about the effects of forcing the body to produce the toxic spike protein. Derek Lowe, an expert in drug development, informed readers:

> If we're causing people to express Spike protein via mRNA or adenovirus vectors, are we damaging them just as if they'd been infected with coronavirus? Fortunately, the answer definitely seems to be "no."
>
> The injection is intramuscular, not into the bloodstream.

Some of the vaccine is going to make it into the blood-stream, of course.

But keep in mind, when the mRNA or adenovirus particles do hit cells outside of the liver or the site of injection, they're still causing them to express Spike protein anchored on their surfaces, not dumping it into the circulation. Here's the EMA briefing document for the Pfizer/BioNTech vaccine—on pages 46 and 47, you can read the results of the distribution studies.[153]

In fact, the Pfizer document Dr. Lowe links to states clearly on page 45:

> No traditional pharmacokinetic or biodistribution studies have been performed with the vaccine candidate BNT162b2.[154]

Eight days after that, the Advisory Committee on Immunization Practices met to discuss the prospect of extending the Emergency Use Authorization of the Pfizer shot to twelve-to-fifteen-year-olds.[155] The trial had enrolled 2,200 youths, split equally between the treatment and placebo groups. Of those, barely half had even as much as two months of follow-up, and little more than a quarter made it to the three-month mark. The researchers determined that the vax elicited levels of antibodies in these youths comparable to those seen in adults. There were sixteen cases of covid reported in patients given placebo, as opposed to three in the treatment arm. None of these cases were severe. There were no deaths.

Five of the youths given the shot suffered serious adverse events, as opposed to two in the placebo arm. The report of the Advisory Committee noted:

> Many of the AEs were reported by a single person. For example, abdominal pain, constipation, and neuralgia was reported by 1 individual. This individual presented with abdominal pain and had multiple physical examinations and

laboratory evaluations for these complaints. Ultimately, a diagnosis of functional abdominal pain was made.

There were also cases of depression and suicidal ideation in the treatment arm, along with one case of depression and anxiety. All of these youths had been on selective serotonin reuptake inhibitors (SSRI's), a class of drugs (including Pfizer's blockbuster drug Zoloft) commonly prescribed for depression. Could these serious adverse events have been due to an interaction between SSRI's and the spike protein? The Advisory Committee seemed remarkably uninterested in finding out.

Then it was the public's turn to speak:

> SAVANNAH STARKEY WHITE: I'd like to honor my son today by speaking about the topic at hand. Baby Remy passed away approximately 12 hours after his CDC recommended schedule at his 2-month appointment. His autopsy came back anaphylactic adverse reaction to the multiple vaccinations received the day prior.
>
> To you, my son was just one baby, but to my children, my husband, and myself—he was our world and it is forever shattered.
>
> Pfizer is filing for the full FDA approval of their covid vaccine this month. It's no secret that the vaccine comes with significant immediate reactions. The list of adverse reactions is growing and the number of complaints are tripling daily. We do not know enough about the long-term effects of this vaccine to approve it for full FDA approval.
>
> Based on the limited study that you all conducted yourselves, 77.4% reported at least 1 systematic reaction. Lymphadenopathy, Bell's palsy, appendicitis, acute myocardial infarction, cerebral vascular accidents were all reported and considered adverse reactions just from your studies alone.

There have been thousands of additional reports to VAERS for serious adverse reactions, blood clots, nerve pain, rashes, hives, multiple deaths, and dozens of others are trickling in. Concerns of infertility are rippling through social media and flooding doctors with concerned patients.

We do not know the long-term effects of this vaccine. We will not know this for 5, 10, or even 20 years. This information is critical and it must be known before the FDA approves it, especially for our children.

JANELLE SULLIVAN: I have a son who is recovered from severe autism. I spoke in front of this panel in the past about how I've recovered him. "Autism, Beyond Despair" was a book that was very helpful. It actually has a chapter as a rebuttal to Paul Offit's book, "Autism's False Prophets." I recovered him doing what Paul Offit says not to do.

Your CDC schedule caused my son to bang his head on cement and to have absence seizures. It is guilty of the worst child abuse on this planet and I seriously fear what your recommendations are going to cause.

You have the power today to say "no." You have the power. It is so much easier for you to do this now than it will be later. You will not be able to take this decision back. It's going to affect so many lives.

These children are not affected from covid. They are affected from your lockdown measures. They are affected from masking, from social distancing, and from not receiving the contact and the love and the hugs and the high-fives that were meant to be given and received.

Our hearts are not meant to be kept separate. They are meant to come together and do great things, and they're also meant to heal, and they don't need you putting all of these poisons in our body.

SUSIE OLSEN CORGAN: One of three of my main issues with this COVID-19 vaccine is the fact that implications of fertility impairment have not been studied, so how can we recommend a vaccine to 12 to 15-year-olds that could potentially cause impairment in their fertility? Why weren't these studies done prior to recommending these vaccines?

According to CDC, it says that we have had a total of 17 deaths in 12-year-olds, 13 in 13-year-olds, 15 in 14-year-olds, and 24 in 15-year-olds. That is a total of 69 deaths that have been attributed to COVID-19 in 12 to 15-year-olds. While the loss of any life is tragic, especially in children, we have to look at this and declare there is no emergency for children in this age range.

How can you, the members of ACIP, who are entrusted with making these decisions, recommend this vaccine based off this data?

All of these words of caution fell upon deaf ears.

On 13 May, the CDC recommended extending emergency use authorization of the covid vaccines to children between the ages of twelve and fifteen, after a fourteen-to-zero vote by its Advisory Committee on Immunization Practices.[156] That same day, an editorial in the *BMJ* questioned the advisability of vaccinating children for the covid. The authors pointed out that children experience only a mild form of covid infection, and that they play only a marginal role in transmitting the disease to others. Indeed, the authors argued, once most adults are vaccinated against the disease, limited circulation of covid among children might in fact be desirable, exposing them to the disease at an age when symptoms are mild, and providing booster re-exposures periodically throughout life as transmission-blocking immunity wanes but disease-blocking immunity remains high.[157]

Again, all of these words of caution fell upon deaf ears.

Four days later, the Vaccine Safety Technical Work Group of the Advisory Committee met to discuss cases of myocarditis following the mRNA shots. The work group concluded that such cases were seen primarily in adolescents and young adults, more often in males than in females, and occurred more often after the second dose than the first dose—again indicating the damage was dose-related. The group concluded that most cases of myocarditis were "mild."[158]

Something like ten to twenty percent of children treated for myocarditis will go on to develop chronic residual heart problems called "dilated cardiomyopathy" and may end up listed for a heart transplant.[159]

The same day, NIAID Director Anthony Fauci appeared as a guest on MSNBC, where he touted the benefits of the mRNA shots:

> We now know that these vaccines are highly, highly effective, number one.
>
> Number two, they're really, really good against variants.
>
> Even if you do get a breakthrough infection, the chances of transmitting it to someone else is exceedingly low.[160]

The next day, a consortium of twenty-five scientists from fifteen different countries issued a manifesto pleading for vigilance regarding the possible harms of the mRNA vaccines:

> COVID-19 encompasses a wide clinical spectrum, ranging from very mild to severe pulmonary pathology and fatal multi-organ disease with inflammatory, cardiovascular, and blood coagulation dysregulation. In this sense, cases of vaccine-related antibody-dependent enhancement or immunopathology would be clinically-indistinguishable from severe COVID-19.

Not a single study has examined the duration of spike protein production in humans following vaccination.

Vaccine-induced Spike synthesis could cause clinical signs of severe COVID-19 and erroneously be counted as new cases of SARS-CoV-2 infections.

Another critical issue to consider given the global nature of SARS-CoV-2 vaccination is autoimmunity. SARS-CoV-2 has numerous immunogenic proteins, and all but one of its immunogenic epitopes have similarities to human proteins.

If vaccination programs worldwide do not institute independent data safety monitoring boards (DSMB), events adjudication committees (EAC), and enact risk mitigation strategies, we will call for a pause in the mass vaccination program.[161]

Again, all of these words of caution fell upon deaf ears.

The next day, British television presenter Piers Morgan offered these words of wisdom on Twitter:

> People who refuse to get jabbed but whine about lockdowns really are a special breed of stupid selfish pr*icks.

Three days later, CNN reported that covid vaccine profits had created nine new billionaires, including the CEO's of both Moderna and BioNTech, with a net worth of about four billion dollars apiece.[162]

Shifting the Goalposts, Again

That same month, the *Merriam-Webster Dictionary*, without any discussion or debate, changed the definition of "vaccine" on its website. The old definition read as follows:

> A preparation of killed microorganisms, living attenuated organisms, or living fully virulent organisms that is adminis-

tered to produce or artificially increase immunity to a particular disease.[163]

This was changed to:

A preparation that is administered—as by injection—to
stimulate the body's immune response against a specific
infectious agent or disease.[164]

The Pfizer shot and the Moderna shot would not even have been
considered vaccines according to the old definition, but they would by the
new one. (And of course, if you change the definition of "vaccine," you
automatically change the definition of "anti-vaxxer," as well.)

A "fact-check" piece in *USA Today* would later confirm all the details
in this story but rated it as "missing context."[165]

The Elephant in the Room

On 1 June, Linda Wastila, Professor of Pharmaceutical Health Services
the University Maryland, along with Peter Doshi, Kim Witczak, David
Healy, and twenty-three other experts, filed a citizen's petition[166] with the
FDA requesting that full approval of the covid vaccines be delayed until a
number of conditions were met:

1) Two years of follow-up of participants originally enrolled in
   clinical trials

2) Substantial evidence of clinical effectiveness that outweighs
   harms in special populations such as infants, children, and
   adolescents; those with past SARS-CoV-2 infection; the
   immunocompromised; pregnant and nursing women; the
   frail elderly; and individuals with cancer, autoimmune disorders, and hematological conditions

3) A thorough assessment of the safety of the spike proteins produced by the body after immunization

4) Completion of vaccine biodistribution studies

5) Thorough investigation of all severe adverse reactions reported following immunization

6) Assessment of safety of individuals receiving more than two doses

7) Inclusion of gene therapy experts in the Vaccines and Related Biological Products Advisory Committee

8) Enforcing stringent conflict-of-interest requirements

The petitioners then went on to explain the reasoning behind each of these requests.

The two-year follow-up period was in fact the length of time proposed by the manufacturers when they registered their Phase III trials of the covid vaccines. The evidence of effectiveness in special populations was requested because risks of vaccination may be higher and/or the risks of covid infection may be lower in many of these, especially the young and those with a previous history of infection by SARS-CoV-2.

Numerous studies had already raised concerns about the safety of the spike protein, which had been linked to a long list of health problems:

- Coagulopathy issues such as blood clots, hemorrhage, thrombocytopenia, heart attacks, and stroke (According to the CDC's Vaccine Adverse Reporting System, or VAERS, as of 1 May there had been 1,222 reports of thrombocytopenia/low platelets and 6,494 reports of blood clots/strokes, including 112 in persons below the age of 25)

- Reproductive issues such as menstrual irregularities, reduced fertility, miscarriages, and preterm births (by then VAERS had received 511 reports of miscarriage and 522 reports of uterine hemorrhage)

- Carcinogenesis

- Transmission of the spike protein to newborns via breast milk

- Neurological disorders such as Guillain-Barré syndrome, acute disseminated encephalomyelitis, meningoencephalomyelitis, encephalitis, encephalopathy, demyelinating disease, and multiple sclerosis

- Autoimmune diseases such as thyroiditis, diabetes mellitus, immune thrombocytopenia, autoimmune hepatitis, primary biliary cholangitis, systemic sclerosis, myasthenia gravis, polymyositis, dermatomyositis, and other inflammatory myopathies

And while both the Pfizer and the Moderna products are intended to be administered in the form of two intramuscular injections, studies submitted by both companies to regulators suggested that the vaccines do not remain near the site of injection but rather distribute widely throughout the body to the liver, brain, heart, lungs, ovaries, testes, and many other places. These studies were not done with the actual vaccines but with similar products. Thus the potential of the covid vaccines to disperse from the point of administration to other parts of the body remained unknown.

Regarding adverse events: the most serious adverse event obviously is death, and as of 1 May 2021, there had been 4,863 deaths associated with the covid vaccines reported to VAERS. We have already noted that these post-marketing reporting systems are generally thought to capture between one and ten percent of all serious adverse events. For calibration, let us also note the swine flu vaccine was taken off the market after five hundred reported cases of Guillain-Barré Syndrome and twenty-five deaths.[167]

There already was evidence that the harms done by these products may be dose-related. Pfizer and Moderna already had indicated that a third dose might be necessary within twelve months, and there was talk of offering these vaccines on an annual basis, like flu shots. The prospect of multiple injections, perhaps as many as seventy in the course of a lifetime, urgently highlighted the need for safety data in individuals receiving more than two doses.

The request for gene therapy experts to be included in the VRBPAC was made in recognition of the fact that these products were of a kind unlike any other vaccine ever before deployed, and in fact met the definition of gene therapy, while the request that analysis of data and decisions regarding any covid vaccine be carried out by experts with no financial relationship to any vaccine manufacturers was made to ensure the independence of the FDA decision-making process from the pecuniary interests of the drugmakers.

The petitioners also argued there were no compelling reasons for the FDA to grant full authorization of the covid vaccines. These products already were available to anyone who wanted them, and the Emergency Use Authorization did not come with an expiration date. To those who were demanding full authorization in order to bolster public confidence in these products, or to justify vaccine mandates, Dr. Wastila and her colleagues replied that they had their priorities backwards, and that such considerations were outside the FDA's brief anyway.

Eight days later, Dr. Wastila, along with Dr. Doshi and Kim Witczak, published a piece in *BMJ Blogs* explaining the reasoning behind the citizens' petition, concluding:

> Finally, regarding the elephant in the room: publicly raising any element of hesitation about covid-19 vaccines will be seen by some as irresponsible, stoking unfounded fears in the public's mind and contributing to the vaccine hesitancy problem trumpeted every day. But the alternatives—privately raising concerns or simply remaining silent—are arguably

more detrimental to public trust in the long run. Staying silent is not the responsible option. [168]

Again, all of these words of caution fell upon deaf ears.

Two days later, Dr. Doshi addressed the FDA Vaccines and Related Biological Products Advisory Committee, arguing there were no grounds for extending the Emergency Use Authorization for COVID-19 vaccines to children.[169] He pointed out that the risk of children contracting covid was tiny, and that the vast majority of those who did experienced only mild symptoms. By contrast, the drugmakers' own trials had shown the rate of adverse events was actually higher in the treatment group than in the placebo group.

Furthermore, he pointed out, there just was not enough known about the long-term harms. Dr. Doshi reminded the committee that the first cases of narcolepsy in adolescents administered the flu vaccines Pandemrix were not noticed until some nine months later, and he referred to the ominous findings regarding the mechanism of action and biodistribution studies already discussed in the citizens' petition filed ten days earlier. He wound up by pointing out the FDA can authorize a product for use in a given population only if benefits outweigh risks for that same population. Whether or not vaccinating children lowers the likelihood of their elders suffering from the covid should not be a consideration.

Again, all of these words of caution fell upon deaf ears.

That same day, Tom Shimabukuro of the Vaccine Safety Team of the CDC Covid-19 Vaccine Task Force reported in a presentation to the Vaccines and Related Biological Products Advisory Committee that VAERS had received 789 reports of myocarditis and pericarditis in children following administration of the covid vaccine. Two hundred and sixteen of these cases occurred after the first shot and 573 after the second—once again indicating a dose-dependent relationship.[170]

The risk of myocarditis and pericarditis was significantly elevated for females between the ages of twelve and twenty-nine years of age and males between twelve and forty-nine—including a staggering thirty-two-fold increase in risk for males between the ages of twelve and seventeen.

Again, all of these words of caution fell upon deaf ears.

On 14 July, Flagship Pioneering (formerly known as Flagship Ventures), the venture capital firm behind Moderna, announced that they had hired former FDA Commissioner Stephen Hahn as Chief Medical Officer. This was six months after the FDA, under Dr. Hahn's leadership, had authorized the Moderna shot for emergency use. Flagship founder and CEO Noubar Afeyan is also Chairman of Moderna.[171]

Two days after that, Pfizer and BioNTech announced their intentions to seek full FDA approval for their products.[172]

They're Killing People

That same day, White House Press Secretary Jen Psaki told reporters:

> We are regularly making sure social media platforms are aware of the latest narratives dangerous to public health that we and many other Americans are seeing across all of social and traditional media.
>
> Let me give you an example. The false narrative remains active out there about COVID-19 vaccines causing infertility—which has been disproven time and time again.[173]

The secretary did not explain how she could have known that, given that we were less than nine months into the vax rollout.

Psaki called for Facebook and other platforms to create "robust enforcement strategies that bridge their properties," adding "You shouldn't be banned from one platform and not others for providing misinformation."

Later that day, President Joseph Biden, as he was preparing to depart for Camp David aboard Marine One, was more succinct. In response to a reporters' question about social media platforms, he replied:

They're killing people.[174]

Five days later, the president appeared on CNN's "Town Hall" meeting hosted by reporter Don Lemon, where he adroitly explained:

> We're not in a position where we think that any virus— including the Delta virus, which is much more transmissible and more deadly in terms of non— unvaccinated people— the vi— the various shots that people are getting now cover that. They're—you're okay. You're not going to—you're not going to get covid if you have these vaccinations.[175]

The next day, an *i24NEWS* report noted that the Health Ministry of Israel (the nation that led the world in the speed and breadth of its vaccine rollout) announced that the efficacy of the Pfizer vax had dropped to a paltry thirty-nine percent as the new Delta variant of the coronavirus surged.[176] In fairness, the piece also noted that the claimed efficacy of the shot against severe COVID-19 remained high, at ninety-one percent, but this begs the question of whether the vax lowers the risk of all serious adverse events. The article also did not mention that cases of severe COVID-19 occurring within four weeks after the first dose were not included in this endpoint.[177]

That same day Israel's health minister lashed out at vaccine refusers, claiming they were putting themselves and the rest of society in danger, and added:

> I have respect for everyone's opinion, but now is not the time to have a debate about vaccines, but to get vaccinated.[178]

Eight days after that, the CDC reported an outbreak of 469 covid cases in Barnstable County, Massachusetts. Three fourths of these occurred among the fully vaccinated, and the great majority of these "breakthrough infections" were symptomatic. PCR testing revealed no difference in viral load between the vaxxed and the unvaxxed.[179]

Screw Your Freedom

The media hate campaign against anti-vaxxers (a category which by now apparently included everyone who had any reservations about any product called a "vaccine") picked up momentum. On 23 July, CNN anchor Don Lemon blasted vaccine skeptics, calling their behavior "idiotic and nonsensical."[180] Four days later, Piers Morgan went further, demanding in a tweet that covid vaccine refusers be denied health care:

> Those who refuse to be vaccinated, with no medical reason not to, should be refused NHS health care if they then catch covid. I'm hearing of anti-vaxxers using up ICU beds in London at vast expense to the taxpayer. Let them pay for their own stupidity and selfishness.

David Olive, business columnist for the *Toronto Star* proclaimed "[Vaccine] passports that prevent mingling of vaccinated and unvaccinated people are the most effective tool we have to prevent a fourth wave."[181] Not to be outdone, author Jessica Valenti, in an op-ed in the *New York Times*, noted that "Gross selfishness masked as American individualism is killing our country and traumatizing our children."[182] And a judge in Hamilton County, New York, ordered a convicted drug offender to get the shot or spend three years in prison.[183]

In fairness, it should be pointed out the authorities provided carrots as well as sticks, demonstrating their tender concern for the immune health of the citizenry by offering free beer, donuts, burgers, fries, and weed in exchange for getting the vax.[184]

On 10 August, former California governor Arnold Schwarzenegger gave an interview on CNN[185] in which he offered the following words of advice:

> There is a virus here. It kills people and the only way we prevent it is: get vaccinated, wear masks, do social distancing,

washing your hands all the time, and not just to think about "Well, my freedom is kind of being disturbed here."

Then the man who had been beloved by millions for his bodybuilding titles, his action movies, and his health and fitness advice looked into the camera and snarled:

Screw your freedom.

Rigorous Scientific Standards

That same day, a Reuters "fact-check" story purported to debunk the claim that mRNA vaccines are gene therapy. The piece quoted several experts but ignored the FDA's own definition, last updated 25 July 2018 and still current at the time of this writing: "Human gene therapy seeks to modify or manipulate the expression of a gene or to alter the biological properties of living cells for therapeutic use."[186]

The piece also neglected to mention that James Smith, CEO of Thomson Reuters until March of 2020 and current Chairman of the Thomson Reuters Foundation, also sits on the Board of Directors of Pfizer.[187]

Six days later, Pfizer and BioNTech filed for FDA approval of a third, booster shot, based on studies that showed the antibody levels waned over time and that the booster increased those levels[188]—without anyone even claiming these heightened antibody levels increased the likelihood of any clinically relevant outcome—and ignoring the unknown potential for harm caused by repeated inundations of the toxic spike protein.

Seven days after that, FDA granted full approval of the Pfizer vax (the two-dose regimen, not the booster shot) for individuals sixteen years and older,[189] without a meeting of the FDA's advisory panel—blatantly ignoring Commissioner Hahn's promise the year before "to use an advisory committee composed of independent experts to ensure deliberations about authorization or licensure are transparent for the public."

Acting FDA Commissioner Janet Woodcock declared:

> The FDA's approval of this vaccine is a milestone as we continue to battle the COVID-19 pandemic. While this and other vaccines have met the FDA's rigorous, scientific standards for emergency use authorization, as the first FDA-approved COVID-19 vaccine, the public can be very confident that this vaccine meets the high standards for safety, effectiveness, and manufacturing quality the FDA requires of an approved product.[190]

Kim Witczak told the *BMJ*:

> These public meetings are imperative in building trust and confidence especially when the vaccines came to market at lightning speed under emergency use authorisation.
>
> The public deserves a transparent process, especially as the call for boosters and mandates are rapidly increasing. These meetings offer a platform where questions can be raised, problems tackled, and data scrutinized in advance of an approval.
>
> It's already concerning that full approval is being based on six months' worth of data despite the clinical trials designed for two years.
>
> There is no control group after Pfizer offered the product to placebo participants before the trials were completed.[191]

Again, all of these words of caution fell upon deaf ears.

In yet another essay in *BMJ Blogs*, Dr. Doshi blasted the FDA decision to grant full approval to the shot.[192] The preprint of Pfizer's trial results had been posted on 28 July and misleadingly titled "Six Month Safety and

Efficacy of the BNT162b2 mRNA COVID-19 Vaccine."[193] In fact, by the data cut-off date of 13 March, only seven percent of trial participants had reached six months of blinded follow-up. In other words, the "up to six months" worth of RCT data was all we were ever going to get—in a trial originally slated to enroll forty-four thousand participants for a full two years.

Dr. Doshi remarked "It is hard to imagine the < 10% of trial participants who remained blinded at six months (which presumably further dwindled after 13 March 2021) could constitute a reliable or valid sample to produce further findings."

The picture emerging from the Moderna trial was equally bleak: by mid-April, ninety-eight percent of the placebo group had gotten the vax.

The lack of long-term follow-up seemed especially egregious in the wake of the specter of waning immunity already beginning to emerge.

Once again all of these words of caution fell upon deaf ears.

The very next day Secretary of Defense Lloyd Austin issued a memorandum mandating that all uniformed service members must get the shot.

That same day, a study by University of Wisconsin researchers cast serious doubt on the ability of the vax to prevent transmission—the linchpin of the justification for vaccine mandates. The researchers found that fully vaxxed asymptomatic subjects were more likely to test positive for COVID-19 and more likely to be shedding the virus.[194]

Two days after that, the organization Public Health and Medical Professionals for Transparency filed a Freedom of Information Act request demanding all the data and information on the vax that had been submitted to the FDA for approval of that product, and in addition demanded expedited processing of their request. PHMPT is an organization which "exists for the sole purpose of disseminating to the public the data and information in the biological product files for each of the COVID-19 vaccines." Among its founders were Peter Doshi, David Healy,

Linda Wastila, and a number of other prominent clinicians, public health experts, and patient advocates, including Aaron Kheriarty, Professor of Psychiatry and Director of Ethics and Public Policy at UC Irvine, and Joseph Ladapo, then Professor of Medicine at UCLA and now Surgeon General of the State of Florida.

In their FOIA request, the petitioners wrote:

> During a time when COVID-19 vaccine mandates are being implemented over the objections of those that have questions about the data and information supporting the safety and efficacy of the Pfizer vaccine, and individuals with those questions are being expelled from employment, school, transportation, and the military, the public has an urgent and immediate need to have access to the data.

I Don't Know What's in It

It was somewhere around this time—no one seems to know exactly when—the following abject statement of self-abnegation began making the rounds on social media:

> I'm fully vaccinated and, no, I don't know what's in it—neither this vaccine, the ones I had as a child, nor in the Big Mac, or hot dogs, or other treatments, whether it's for cancer, AIDS, the one for polyarthritis, or vaccines for infants or children.
>
> I also don't know what's in Ibuprofen, Paracetamol, or other meds, it just cures my headaches & my pains.
>
> I don't know what's in the ink for tattoos, vaping, Botox and fillers, or every ingredient in my soap or shampoo or even deodorants. I don't know the long-term effect of mobile phone use or whether or not that restaurant I just ate at REALLY used clean foods and washed their hands.

In short...

There's a lot of things I don't know and never will...

I just know one thing: life is short, very short, and I still want to do something other than just going to work every day or staying locked in my home. I still want to travel and hug people without fear and find a little feeling of life "before."

As a child and as an adult I've been vaccinated for mumps, measles, polio, chickenpox, and quite a few others; my parents and I trusted the science and never had to suffer through or transmit any of the said diseases and,

I'm vaccinated, not to please the government but:

- To not die from Covid-19
- To NOT clutter a hospital bed if I get sick
- To hug my loved ones
- To not have to do PCR or antigenic tests to go to a restaurant, go on holidays, and many more things to come
- To live my life
- To see and hug my family and friends
- For Covid-19 to be an old memory
- To protect us

If the goal of lockdowns, school closures, masking, fear messaging, vaccine passports, endless testing, and the like was to break the will of the citizenry, crush their spirit, and induce them to accede to having anything at all shot into their bodies as long as it is called a "vaccine," all this seems to have succeeded—at least in some of us.

Let Them Die

The front-page headline of the 26 August issue of the *Toronto Star* read "Simmering Divide Over Who Isn't Vaccinated,"[195] and the cover featured these bons mots culled from Twitter:

"If an unvaccinated person catches [covid] from someone who is vaccinated, too bad."

"I have no empathy left for the unvaccinated. Let them die."

"Unvaccinated patients do not deserve ICU beds."

"At this point, who cares. Stick the unvaccinated in a tent outside and tend to them when the staff has time."

In the accompanying story, the *Star* took the high road, dispensing soothing platitudes about the need for empathy, and quoting an expert who noted that many of the covid vaccine skeptics are not "staunch anti-vaxxers," but rather are "victims of misinformation or systemic barriers, like not having access to a family doctor to answer questions about the safety of vaccines."

The possibility that anyone might have rational grounds for avoiding the shots was not considered.

Shifting the Goalposts—Yet Again

On the first day of September, the CDC followed the lead of the *Merriam-Webster Dictionary* and changed its definition of "vaccine" on its website. Prior to 2015, the word was defined as "Injection of a killed or weakened infectious organism in order to prevent disease." In 2015 that definition was changed to this rather vague formulation: "The act of introducing a vaccine into the body to produce immunity to a specific disease."

In the wake of mounting evidence of waning antibody levels in double-vaxxed subjects, that definition was changed once again, to the even more vague "Act of introducing a vaccine into the body to protect against a specific disease."

The covid shots may qualify as a vaccine under this definition, but these criteria are so vague that any substance taken prophylactically for any ailment—quinine, antibiotics, aspirin—could now be considered a "vaccine."

An Associated Press "fact-check" would later confirm all this, but denied this had anything to do with waning antibody levels in recipients of the covid vaccines. Again, the story was rated as "missing context."[196]

I Understand Your Anger

Four days after the CDC changed its definition of "vaccine," Dr. Fauci claimed in an interview with CNN that intensive care units in many parts of the country were approaching full capacity, predicting "You're going to be in a situation where you're going to have to make some tough choices." Fauci said he doubted that vaccination status would be used in determining who gets an ICU bed, but added ominously "There's talk of that."[197]

Late-night comedian Jimmy Kimmel offered this clever commentary:

> That choice doesn't seem so tough to me. Vaccinated person having a heart attack? Yes, come right in, we'll take care of you. Unvaccinated guy who gobbled horse goo? Rest in peace, Wheezy.[198]

Not to be outdone, on 7 September,[199] washed-up radio shock jock Howard Stern treated listeners to this soliloquy:

> When are we gonna stop putting up with the idiots in this country and just say it's mandatory to get vaccinated? Fuck 'em. Fuck their freedom.

To the "imbeciles" who refused the shot and found themselves hospitalized, Stern had this to say:

Go fuck yourself. You had the cure and you wouldn't take it.

Two days later, former Baltimore City Health Commissioner and CNN Medical Analyst Leana Wen sided with these distinguished experts, telling viewers:

> We need to start looking at the choice to remain unvaccinated the same as we look at driving while intoxicated.
>
> The vaccinated should not have to pay the price for the so-called choices of the unvaccinated anymore.[200]

That same day, President Biden ordered federal workers and contractors to get the vax, and for all employers with over one hundred workers to require either vaccinations or weekly testing.[201] Members of Congress and their staffs were exempted from this executive order.[202]

The president told the nation:

> My message to unvaccinated Americans is this: what more is there to wait for? What more do you need to see? We have made vaccinations free, safe, & convenient. The vaccine is FDA approved. Over 200 million Americans have gotten at least one shot. We have been patient, but our patience is wearing thin, and the refusal has cost all of us.
>
> To the vaccinated, I understand your anger towards the vaccinated.

In all of my sixty years on this earth, I had never heard a president of the United States of America address the citizenry in such a menacing fashion. Never.

Six days later, CNN reporter Don Lemon deftly put to rest people's irrational fears about the covid vaccines:

> People talk about "Well, I don't know what's in the shot. I don't know what's in that shot." You know what they get shots

in nowadays? In their rear ends. They're getting shots to make it bigger. They're getting shots in their face. They don't know what's in Botox. They don't know what's in the stuff—nothing wrong with Botox. Look, I tried it once. My eyebrow went up. I don't have it now. As you can see, I got all these wrinkles. Everybody asks me "When are you going to get Botox?" But listen—nothing wrong with Botox. Do people really know what's in stuff that they inject in their bodies all the time? What they eat? What they drink? Stop it! Stop it with the ignorance![203]

Lemon did not mention that almost exactly a year before, his employer had received a $3.6 million donation from the Bill and Melinda Gates Foundation,[204] which in turn has invested heavily in vaccine manufacturers, including Pfizer and BioNTech.[205] Although, in fairness, it should be pointed out that a 2016 study found little evidence of explicit editorial review of media content by not-for-profit funding organizations such as the Bill and Melinda Gates Foundation.[206]

That study was funded by the Bill and Melinda Gates Foundation.

Real-World Efficacy

Meanwhile, the same day President Biden delivered his words of warning to the unvaccinated, the FDA denied expedited processing of the PHMPT request for the Pfizer data. One week later, PHMPT filed suit in the Northern District Court of Texas.

Six days after that, the FDA authorized a third (booster) dose of the Pfizer shot for individuals aged sixty-five and older, as well as individuals between the ages of eighteen and sixty-four who were judged to be at high risk for severe COVID-19, or whose frequent institutional or occupational exposure puts them at risk for serious complications of COVID-19.[207]

On the last day of September, a study by Harvard scientists cast serious doubt on the efficacy of the vaccine in real-world conditions. The researchers examined data from sixty-eight different nations and 2,947 US counties and found no correlation between vaccine coverage and new cases of COVID-19. Indeed, the nation-level analysis found a slight (although not statistically significant) positive correlation between vaccination coverage and infection rates.[208]

The researchers went on to note some further seemingly anomalous results arising from their analysis. Israel, with sixty percent of its population fully vaxxed, had the highest rate of new covid cases, and that Iceland and Portugal, each with vaccination rates of over seventy-five percent, had higher infection rates than either Viet Nam or South Africa, where the rate of vaccination was around ten percent. And when they looked at the five US counties where vaccination rates were highest, they found four of the five had been identified by the CDC as "high-transmission" counties.

Rather than follow these startling findings to their obvious conclusion—that if we stopped vaccinating people for covid we probably wouldn't notice any difference—the authors wrapped things up with a declaration of fealty to the covid vaccines.

Mavericks and Misfits

That same day, Dr. Breggin (along with his wife, Ginger Ross Breggin) released their new book, *COVID-19 and the Global Predators: We Are the Prey*.[209] The book covered not just the mendacity of the vaccine manufacturers but also the inflated death toll attributed to the pandemic, the destruction wrought by lockdowns, the uselessness of masks, the suppression of safe and effective early-stage treatments shown to keep patients alive and out of hospital, the death toll that followed a governor's decision to place thousands of patients with fulminating illness into nursing homes, and much more—it was all there, his most magnificent work, the culmination of a lifetime of evaluating medical information, comforting the afflicted, and speaking truth to power.

In the preface the authors issued this exhortation:

> Seekers of liberty and seekers of truth, rebels, individual-
> ists, explorers, cowboys, artists, nonconformists, intellectuals,
> mavericks, misfits, professionals, Divergents, free thinkers,
> and people of faith—even establishment members who now
> see the light—all of us must stand together. We have only
> ourselves. We must with true grit and respect and grace forge
> ahead and create a new tomorrow.
>
> You will find yourself no longer alone. You will become
> empowered. You will make wonderful new friends. Your
> life will take on new meaning when you realize you have a
> rare opportunity in history to fight for Western values, the
> Judeo-Christian traditions, and the existence of individual
> and political liberty on earth.

We Are Never Going to Learn How Safe This Vaccine Is Until We Start Giving It

On 6 October, Pfizer submitted to the FDA its application for Emergency Use Authorization of the shot for children five through eleven years of age, to be administered in the form of two intramuscular injections, ten micrograms apiece instead of the thirty micrograms given to adolescents and adults.

Two weeks later, the FDA granted full approval to a third (booster) shot of the Moderna vaccine for certain populations—again, in the wake of mounting evidence of waning immunity after two injections.[210]

Six days after that, the Vaccines and Related Biological Products Advisory Committee met to discuss approving the Pfizer shot for five-to-eleven-year-olds.[211] The trial looked at two cohorts of patients. The first cohort enrolled 1,518 patients in the treatment group and 750 in the placebo arm, with a minimum of two months of follow-up. The second cohort contained 1,591 patients in the treatment arm and 788 in the placebo arm. Median follow-up time for this cohort was a mere seventeen days.

There were three cases of COVID-19 in the treatment group as opposed to sixteen among those given placebo. There were no cases of severe covid in either arm of the trial, and no deaths.

The most interesting part of the FDA briefing document was Table 14, which modeled the number of hospitalizations for both covid and myocarditis per million vaccinated patients, under a variety of starting assumptions. The model predicted that vaccinating one million five-to-eleven-year-olds would prevent anywhere from seven to sixty-two covid ICU admissions—at the cost of an additional twenty-nine to fifty-eight ICU admissions for myocarditis.

In other words, according to the FDA, the number of ICU admissions prevented by the shot would be almost exactly equal to the number caused by the shot.

And even these underwhelming numbers were based on the assumption that none of the kiddies who got the vax had pre-existing immunity to the covid—an absolutely indefensible supposition.

So why grant approval? Eric Rubin, Professor of Immunology and Infectious Diseases at the Harvard T.H. Chan School of Public Health, Associate Physician at Brigham and Young Women's Hospital, and Editor-in-Chief of the New England Journal of Medicine, told the FDA panel:

> We are never going to learn how safe this vaccine is unless we start giving it.[212]

The same day New York City Mayor Bill de Blasio announced that all municipal workers would be required to get the shot by 29 October or face the loss of their jobs.[213]

Three days later, the Pfizer vax was authorized for emergency use in children.[214]

* * *

In summary: there was no compelling reason for the FDA to grant full approval to the Pfizer shot—under the Emergency Use Authorization, the shot was already available to anyone who wanted it—and lots of reasons to hold off, given the complete lack of long-term safety data, the number of participants who dropped out of the trial for "protocol violations," the mounting toll of serious adverse events and deaths reported to VAERS, the lack of data regarding the biodistribution of the mRNA vaccine, concerns over the toxic effects of the spike protein, waning immunity in vaccine recipients, and much more.

We were warned of all this by eminently credentialed experts writing in the pages of the world's most prestigious medical journal.

But the FDA granted full approval anyway.

How did all this work out for us?

CHAPTER FIVE

Standing Up to Tyranny

November–December 2021

We Are Not Anecdotes

Telling the truth in today's cancel culture is not necessarily easy. You can pay a pretty heavy price for it.

So said Senator Ron Johnson of Wisconsin at the opening of the meeting of the Expert Panel on Federal Vaccine Mandates held at the Russell Senate Office Building on Tuesday 2 November 2021.

I attended the meeting, along with a motley assortment of free-lance journalists, bloggers, patient advocates, and their families. The meeting had been organized by Peter Doshi, Linda Wastila, David Healy, and Kim Witczak, all four of whom describe themselves as true-blue Democrats. Senator Johnson, at whose behest the meeting was organized, is a Republican.

Conspicuous by their absence were NIH Director Francis Collins, NIAID Director Anthony Fauci, and the CEO's of Pfizer, Moderna, and BioNTech, all of whom had been invited to attend. None of them accepted.

Also conspicuous by their absence were any representatives from the legacy media.

Looking every bit the part of a United States senator—tall, white-haired, imperially slim—Johnson kicked off the proceedings by referring to President Biden's recent pronouncement that "this is an epidemic of the unvaccinated," adding "I wish that were true," and going on to point out that in the United Kingdom, sixty-three percent of those who died of the covid were fully vaccinated.

Senator Johnson decried the forced vaccination of doctors and nurses, "the heroes of covid" who risked their health and lives treating patients and now are being threatened with the loss of their livelihoods for not getting the shot—even the ones who had already contracted the disease and now had robust, long-lasting natural immunity.

The senator then introduced Brianne Dressen, a wife, mother, and preschool teacher turned patient advocate after she enrolled in a vaccine trial and her health was destroyed by the vax. (Brianne had received the Astra-Zeneca vaccine, which like the Pfizer and the Moderna shots forces the body to manufacture the spike protein, but which unlike these nostrums inserts DNA into the cells rather than RNA. This product is not generally available in the United States.)

Brianne had this to say:

> We are everyday Americans. We are Republicans, Democrats, Independents. This is not political. This is a human issue.

After receiving the shot, Brianne suffered a cascade of neurological symptoms. "I feel like I'm being electrocuted, 24–7," she said.

"At first I thought I was alone," she told the audience. "I found there were thousands like me."

Seventy percent of the covid vaccine injury victims she had spoken to had no pre-existing health conditions, and ninety-four percent had no problems with any other vaccine they had received. The vast majority of them had received all the recommended vaccines, including the flu shot.

> We reached out to academics. None of them can get their research published. We reached out to the media. We were told "We can't do anything to make the vaccine look bad."
>
> We are completely on our own.
>
> All we have is each other.
>
> We have been branded as anti-vaxxers. We had our Facebook groups pulled apart. I have lost contact with Facebook friends who were on the verge of suicide.

Dressen's testimony was followed by that of a number of distinguished researchers and clinicians who decried the lack of access to the data and the speed at which the vaccines were rushed to the market. Dr. Wastila addressed the panel as follows:

> We know absolutely nothing about the long-term harms of these vaccines.
>
> We barely know anything about the immediate harms.
>
> We're not opposed to vaccines. We're opposed to their mandated use.

Regarding herself and her fellow panel members, she had this to say:

> We are citizens who have done our civic duty but when we experience serious adverse effects we were left high and dry by FDA, CDC, the NIH, and medical professionals. We are scientists alarmed by the toxic environment in academia and scientific publishing. We are military leaders concerned about vaccine safety in the armed services. We are clinicians who want to treat patients harmed by vaccines but whose practices are limited by their employers and professional boards. And we are lawyers and patient advocates seeking help for our

injured clients and their families. We are the people you haven't heard from.

And we have nothing, absolutely nothing to gain from being here. Indeed, we have everything to lose, including our jobs, our titles, our livelihoods. But we don't intend to go away until we see some real change.

Lieutenant Colonel Theresa Long, Surgeon for the US Army's First Aviation Brigade, deplored the haste with which the vaccines had been brought to market. Noting that the entire US military has lost only twelve soldiers to covid, she declared "We're going to risk the entire fighting force for a vaccine with two months of safety data."

"These are soldiers, not lab rats," she added angrily.

Dr. Long went on to recount her own experience working with Air Force pilots suffering from vaccine injuries:

> I saw five patients in clinic, two of which presented with chest pain, days to weeks after vaccination, and were subsequently diagnosed with pericarditis and worked up to rule out myocarditis. The third pilot had been vaccinated and felt like he was drunk, chronically fatigued twenty-four hours after vaccination. The pilot told me he didn't know what to do so he drank a lot of coffee to try and, quote, wake himself up, and continued to fly until he realized it wasn't going away.
>
> After I reported to my command my concerns that in one morning I had to ground three out of three pilots due to vaccine injuries, the next day my patients were canceled, my charts were pulled for review, and I was told I would not be seeing acute patients anymore.

She went on to point out that it took forty years for the full toxic effects of the anti-miscarriage drug diethylstilbesterol, including infertility and ovarian cancer, to become apparent—and that these effects continued to manifest themselves two generations down the road.

"There is no substitute for time," Dr. Long told the audience.

In addition, the audience heard directly from more patients whose lives were turned upside-down by the vax. One by one they recounted how they (or their loved ones) took the shot, in good faith, and suffered devastating consequences.

Kyle Warner was a professional mountain bike racer and three-time national champion. After getting the vax he developed pericarditis and Postural Orthostatic Tachycardia Syndrome (POTS), and ended up bedridden.

"I fear that my career has officially ended," he told the panel.

Suzanna Newell of Saint Paul, Minnesota was a triathlete until she was vaccinated: "I aged forty years in one night," she recalled. Twelve-year-old Maddie de Garay of Cincinnati, Ohio was enrolled in the Pfizer trial and suffered dizziness, tachycardia, and chest pains; she ended up in a wheelchair and dependent on a feeding tube. The only adverse event listed for her in the published trial data was "functional abdominal pain." Her brother was also enrolled in the same trial; he happened to be in the placebo arm and escaped unscathed.

And Ernest Ramirez of Austin, Texas, testified:

> I was the father of a sixteen-year-old. I was a single parent. I got the vaccine to protect my son.
>
> Me and my son, we were never apart—always together. I always said "It was you and me against the world."

The younger Ramirez had big dreams. He joined the Junior ROTC program in his high school and planned to enlist in the United States Air Force. He got the vax as well, after the FDA declared it safe and effective for youths. The young man subsequently collapsed and died while playing basketball with his friends.

My government lied to me. They said it was safe. Now I go
home to an empty house.

Holding up a picture of his son's coffin, Ernest told the audience "Don't
make the same mistake I did."

Brianne Dressen addressed the panel once more. She noted that while
Astra-Zeneca had promised to pay all the medical expense of subjects who
were injured in the course of the trials, she was dropped from the trial
and the company cut off all communication with her—missing out on ten
months' worth of safety data. Meanwhile, she told the panel, she and her
husband have had to re-finance their home in order to pay for her medical
expenses.

Brianne went on to read from a letter she received from a fellow covid
vaccine injury sufferer:

I cannot take this any longer.
This has taken everything away from me.
This is beyond the worst torture.
Please accept my apologies.
I must bid farewell to the world.
Please tell our stories.
Goodbye my friend.

Then Senator Johnson called on Aditi Bhargava, Professor Emeritus in
the Biomedical Sciences Graduate Program at the University of California
at San Francisco. A slight woman with long wavy dark hair, Dr. Bhargava
spoke with quiet authority as twelve-year-old Maddie de Garay tossed and
turned beneath her blanket, on her cot placed behind the distinguished
expert:

Thank you for the invitation. My name is Aditi Bhargava. I'm
a professor at UCSF and a molecular biologist with thirty-
three years of research experience,

Natural immunity is the gold standard. CDC estimates that nearly forty percent of the country is already infected with SARS-CoV-2 and thus naturally immune. And that was all before the more transmissible Delta variant took hold.

Living in a bubble or sterile conditions is counterproductive to everything we know about strengthening the immune system. It's Immunology 101. To downplay the protective powers of our immune system goes against the founding principles of immunology.

Several studies about SARS-CoV-2 are validating that knowledge. There is no documented case of a naturally immune person getting infected with severe disease or hospitalization. In sharp contrast, there are thousands of cases of severe covid hospitalizations and deaths in fully vaccinated people.

CDC now estimates the ninety percent of Americans over the age of sixteen now have antibodies against SARS-CoV-2. But vaccine-induced antibodies are only a small fraction of immune responses. New studies from the British Health Ministry suggest that covid vaccines might interfere with the ability of our immune system to produce antibodies against other parts of the virus—crucial aspect for developing protection.

The spike antibodies are incomplete and cherry-picked stories. Vaccine-induced protection fell to between thirty-three percent and forty-two percent within two months. It should not have taken the Massachusetts breakthrough infections in the summer to discover that fully vaccinated people are just as vulnerable to being infected and transmit SARS-CoV-2 as the unvaccinated.

If all we can do is prevent symptoms and severe disease, we should be talking about drugs which treat covid, not vaccines and mandates. We lost the opportunity of discovering these major shortcomings by torpedoing the clinical trials, and placebo groups were eliminated just two months after the second dose. Instead, we are learning through trials and errors on hundreds of millions of people.

And we insist on eliminating a very important control group by these vaccine mandates. There is no scientific study or experimental design in which we can learn anything of value without a control group. Certainly not about safety and efficacy.

Persistent high levels of antibodies often indicate pathology to the body's immune system. That is the basis of autoimmune disease. Hence boosters' long-term adverse events should be weighed seriously.

The notion that we are in an emergency nearly two years into the pandemic and that should justify cutting corners or taking shortcuts is simply wrong. Trust in scientific method is at stake.

Next slide, please.

Media reports often state "the science is clear." But scientific publications do not claim the science is clear. And as you have heard from various testimonies, real people suffered serious adverse events and perhaps lifelong disabilities due to the sloppy trials.

I will conclude by asking you, If the vaccines don't prevent infection or transmission, surely mandating vaccinating person A to protect person B is pointless. But if the vaccines are effective in preventing infection and transmission, decrease symptoms, hospitalization rates and death, then what do the vaccinated fear?

The meeting also featured a message from Dr. Healy, who testified by video owing to his refusal to travel as long as the vaccine mandates for travelers were in place. He began with these words:

> I am a doctor who treats patients. I also am one of the few people you will ever meet who has seen the actual case records from a company clinical trial.

Dr. Healy went on to discuss some particularly egregious examples of the way drug companies hide the harms in their trials. He mentioned one case in which a participant's death was recorded as "death by burning," neglecting to mention the patient had poured gasoline on himself and set himself on fire. In another case, a patient who took GlaxoSmithKline blockbuster drug Paxil and ended up threatening people with a gun had been coded as "intercurrent illness." He also discussed the sad sordid tale of Matt Miller, whom we learned about in a previous chapter.

Dr. Healy concluded with these words:

> Our job as media people or doctors is to make sense of the story the person in front of us is telling—does it make sense that a drug or vaccine caused this or is some fanciful explanation more likely.
>
> I have interviewed all the people injured by vaccines you will hear from here today and stand behind their hunch that it has been the vaccine that has caused what you will hear them tell you.
>
> Data are the bedrock of science. Bri, Maddie and everyone you have heard from are the data—anything short of the full person is not the real thing. You need to be able to cross-examine them and me. Sure, your view of what is

wrong will be provisional—but this is what scientific views are—provisional.

It is not science if you can't see the data. No one sees Pfizer RCT data—not even FDA. You have to be able to see people like Bri and Maddie, who were in RCTs, and see if you agree with their story or agree with Pfizer's fairy tale that there were no serious vaccine related adverse events in their trials.

Pfizer don't do science. They do business. FDA know and enable this. Accepting mandates without data, opens the door to Tyranny.

Then it was Dr. Doshi's turn to speak:

We're told to keep following the science. What we're following is not a scientific process based on open data. We're following a process in which the data are treated as secret. And in my view there's something very unscientific about that.

The point I'm trying to make is fairly simple. The data for covid vaccines isn't available and it won't be available for years. Yet we are not just asking, but mandating millions of people take these products. Whatever word you want to use to describe this situation, without data, it's not science.

After Dr. Doshi had his say, Kim Witczak took to the microphone. Kim recounted the story of her husband Woody's suicide after taking Zoloft, then added:

I would have thought the FDA would have wanted to get to the bottom of what was going on. But FDA officials instead told us, Oh, these stories—a.k.a. my life—are just anecdotes.

Initially I thought this was just an isolated incident with antidepressants. Soon I realized it was a bigger systemic problem with our nation's drug safety system, a system driven by commercial interests and compounded by issues such as lack of transparency, conflict of interest, undue influence, and politics within the FDA and CDC.

And then there's just the plain sad fact that most people just prefer to talk about the benefits of the drugs. The side effects or harms—that's a downer. Ignorance is bliss—until you're the one it impacts.

When the state and federal governments began to push this mass vaccination program, I followed the situation with great interest. Trumpeted as safe and effective, the vaccines were positioned as the only way out of this pandemic. If you dared to question the science, the safety, or public narrative, you were censored or labeled as spreading misinformation, or called an anti-vaxxer.

As a member of another FDA advisory committee, I can tell you that almost every new drug that we are reviewing in the recent years has come to us using a fast-tracking mechanism—much like the EUA track of the vaccine. The FDA priority is to approve drugs, and get 'em on the market quickly, with limited trial data. Safety is usually considered after the fact.

Finally I want to briefly touch on mandates that are affecting all of our lives. This is not a red or a blue issue. This is a human rights issue. Where there's risk, there must also be choice.

People should not be coerced or bribed to choose between their freedom to bodily autonomy or their livelihood and being injected. This is a human rights/social justice issue. Public health may be a population-based approach, but we need to remember we are treating individuals, and a one-size-fits-all does not always work.

People dismiss harms as rare. Well, when you are the person who is harmed, it is your hundred percent. It is your reality.

Unfortunately I hear from people every day that learned this the hard way. They wished they knew of the potential risk before their lives were forever altered. No one should ever have to ask, after the fact, How come I didn't know?

We are not anecdotes.

Helter-Skelter

That same day, an article in the *BMJ* by investigative reporter Paul Thacker reported a whistleblower had revealed numerous irregularities at one of the contract research centers charged with testing the Pfizer shot for safety and effectiveness.[215]

The whistleblower, Brook Jackson, was described as a trained clinical trial auditor with fifteen years' experience in clinical research coordination and management. During the eighteen days she was employed by Ventavia Research Group in Texas, she observed numerous safety and protocol violations, including the following:

- Needles discarded in a plastic biohazard bag instead of instead of a sharps box

- Vaccine packaging materials with trial participants' identification numbers written on them left in the open, potentially unblinding the participants

- Drug assignment information printouts left in participants' medical charts, potentially unblinding clinicians

- Participants placed in hallways after injections and not monitored by clinical staff (a rare but potentially lethal complication of any vaccine is syncope or fainting, which, on rare occasions, has resulted in fatal head injury)

- Lack of timely follow-up on patients who experienced adverse events

- Protocol deviations not reported

- Mislabeled laboratory specimens

- Lack of enough employees to swab all participants with "covid-like symptoms" to detect presence of symptomatic COVID-19, the trial's primary endpoint

- Retaliation against staff members who reported problems

After repeatedly notifying her superiors of these problems, Jackson took her concerns to the FDA and was fired by Ventavia the same day. She said this was the only time she had been fired during her twenty-year career in research. Jackson had provided the *BMJ* with photos, company documents, audio recordings, and emails to back up her claims.

The *BMJ* interviewed other former Ventavia employees as well, who corroborated many of Jackson's claims. One said she had worked on over four dozen clinical trials but had never encountered such a "helter-skelter" environment as she found at Ventavia.

According to the article, only nine of the trial's 153 sites had been inspected by the FDA. Ventavia was not among them.

Eight days later, the "fact-checking" website Lead Stories published an article titled "Fact Check: The British Medical Journal Did NOT Reveal Disqualifying and Ignored Reports of Flaws in Pfizer COVID-19 Vaccine Trials."[216] The piece did not refute a single assertion made in the *BMJ* article but instead proceeded to kick over one straw man after another:

Medical experts say the claims aren't serious enough to discredit data from the clinical trials, which is what Pfizer and the FDA say they concluded.

Ventavia managed 3 of 153 sites at which the trial was carried out.

Pfizer says it has reviewed the claims and found them to be unproven.

On Twitter, Jackson does not express unreserved support for covid vaccines.

That last pronouncement was particularly bizarre. Since when does any citizen have an obligation to express "unreserved support" for anything?

I asked Dr. Healy how concerned we should be about the kinds of problems reported by Jackson. Here is what he had to say:

Part of the problem here for me is that people don't realize how drug company trials function. There's a lot of shoddy practice and for years there's been invention of patients that don't exist. There's been things going on that are worse than some of the things Brook reports on.

So from that point of view, what she's saying is clearly bad and clearly compromises the results that come out of the trial. But it's no worse than a lot of what's been happening in drug trials over the course of the last two or three decades. So we can say, Well, we should be awfully worried about the mRNA trials, but we should have been awfully worried about the drug trials before that, and have somehow managed to turn a blind eye to them. And I would imagine most people are doing the same thing as regards the mRNA trials, just turning a blind eye to it, and that includes the FDA.

On 18 November, Reuters reported that the FDA had filed court papers regarding the PHMPT request for the Pfizer trial data. Despite having over eighteen thousand employees and an annual budget of $6.5 billion, the agency argued it should be expected to produce no more than five hundred pages of data per month. At that rate, it was estimated, it would take the FDA fifty-five years to release all the trial data[217] Less than a month later, this estimate was revised upwards to seventy-five years.[218]

The FDA had granted full approval of the Pfizer shot after taking just 108 days to review the same documents.

A Winter of Severe Illness and Death

Three days later, the FDA extended the Emergency Use Authorization of a booster shot for both the Pfizer and the Moderna vaccines to all adults between the ages of eighteen and sixty-four.[219] The FDA made this decision without convening a meeting of its advisory panel.[220]

Five days after that, the World Health Organization designated the new B.1.1.529 variant, first encountered a few days earlier in Botswana and South Africa, a "variant of concern." This new variant was christened "Omicron."[221]

On the first day of December, the first case of Omicron was reported in the United States, and by 8 December eight cases had been recorded in twenty-two states.[222] This new variant would prove to be both more transmissible and less virulent than its predecessors—exactly what we would expect to happen as the virus continued to evolve.

On 9 December, Emergency Use Authorization of the booster shot was extended to sixteen- and seventeen-year-olds as well.[223] Again this decision was made without convening a meeting of the advisory panel.[224]

That same day President Biden warned the nation:

> We are looking at a winter of severe illness and death for the unvaccinated -- for themselves, their families and the hospitals they'll soon overwhelm. But there's good news: If you're

vaccinated and you have your booster shot, you're protected from severe illness and death.[225]

The next day, *BMJ* editors Fiona Goodlee and Kamran Abbasi published an "open letter" to Mark Zuckerberg, CEO of Facebook.[226] After noting the 2 November piece by Thacker was published following "Legal review, external peer review, and subject to The *BMJ*'s usual high level editorial oversight and review," they went on to claim that from 10 November, readers began reporting a variety of problems when trying to share the article. Some were unable to share at all, while others had their posts flagged "Missing Context... Independent Fact-Checkers say this information could mislead people" and were warned that sharing the article would result in having their posts moved lower in the feed.

After pointing out the Lead Stories article failed to mention even a single factual error in the piece, the two editors asked Zuckerberg to act swiftly to remove the "fact-checking" label and the link to the Lead Stories article, and allow readers to share the story freely. They also requested that the CEO "generally to reconsider and review your investment in and approach to fact checking as well."

The next day, Lead Stories published their reply to the open letter.[227] Again, they failed to point out a single factual error in the original *BMJ* piece, and then went on to accuse the editors of publishing the story under a "scare headline," adding that Jackson was "not a lab-coated scientist titrating doses or checking symptoms," dismissed her credentials as "a 30-hour certification in auditing techniques" (ignoring her twenty years' experience in the field), and added ominously:

> When the U.S. 5th Circuit Court of Appeals ruled against a federal employee vaccine mandate, she tweeted "HUGE!" **and not with a frowny emoji.** [Emphasis added]

A Bitter Dispute

The same day the *BMJ* open letter came out, the *New York Times* reported that Moderna and the NIH had become embroiled in a bitter dispute over the key patent for the Moderna shot.[228] The patent application, filed the previous July, left off the names of three NIH investigators who were said to have played an essential role in the development of the vax.

The application concerned the DNA sequence for the spike protein. Moderna and the NIH had been working together on coronaviruses for four years before the pandemic struck, so collaborating on the vaccine for the new pathogen seemed like the logical next step. Two teams working in parallel, one from Moderna and one from the NIH, had come up with the exact same genetic sequence. But, Moderna's lawyers said, only Moderna scientists deserved credit for the discovery.

The article noted that Moderna had received $1.4 billion from the federal government to develop and test its vaccine and another $8.1 billion to provide the country with half a billion doses, and that the company stood to make $35 billion from its discovery by the end of 2022. A commentary in *Nature* predicted the dispute could go all the way to the Supreme Court, and drag on for years and years.[229]

On 6 December, NYC Mayor Bill de Blasio announced he was extending the covid vaccine mandate to private-sector workers.[230]

Sheer Stupidity

Meanwhile, the media hate campaign against covid vaccine skeptics continued. On 21 November, Piers Morgan tweeted:

> Imagine being scared of having a safe, well-regulated, 4-second vaccine shot, when previous generations braved gun shots for years on end to save us from tyranny?
>
> Antivaxxers really are a bunch of spineless pussies.

On 8 December, in an op-ep piece in the *New York Times*, Charles M. Blow fired off this salvo:

> Call me one of the intolerant. That's what I am. I will not coddle willful ignorance anymore.[231]

Not to be outdone, grossly obese British television presenter Andrew Neil served up this diatribe:

> There are still 5 million unvaccinated British adults, who through fear, ignorance, irresponsibility, or sheer stupidity refuse to be jabbed. In doing so, they endanger not just themselves but the rest of us.[232]

Five days later, the following headline ran in the *Evening Standard*:

> The Unvaccinated Have Become a Lethal Liability We Can Ill-Afford[233]

Five days after that, Piers Morgan offered this modest proposal on Twitter:

> Footballers who refuse to be jabbed should be refused treatment for injuries. After all, why should they trust doctors about treatment for broken legs & torn ligaments if they don't trust them about a life-saving vaccine?

Two days later, the famous television personality followed up with this witty commentary:

> Anti-vaxxers will inevitably prolong the pandemic, thus curbing the very freedom they keep shrieking about for longer than if they all just stopped being gigantic babies and took a little prick in their arms.

The next day, Brown University economics professor Emily Oster chimed in, trying to cast herself as the voice of sweet reason:

> Shaming people who haven't gotten vaccinated is not likely to work at this point (or ever).
>
> What will?
>
> Individual family pressure: Maybe.
>
> Vaccine requirements for things you want to do (domestic air/train travel, work, sports events): Yes.

I Am Struggling to Understand

On Christmas Eve, the *BMJ* published an essay titled "I Am Struggling to Understand Why Patients Decide Not to Get the Covid Vaccine."[234] The anonymous author had this to say:

> In my career I have treated hundreds of patients who are in hospital because of choices they have made; smokers, skiers injured on the slopes, along with patients who have inserted various objects into their orifices not intended for the purpose. I have never felt judgemental. I understand it is their right to choose, and while I may not agree with their choices, my job is to treat them with compassion, but not judgement. I have never found that difficult.
>
> Until now. I am struggling to understand why patients decide not to get the covid vaccine. I see patient after patient on the labour ward, in emergency theatre, and in intensive care who have chosen not to have the vaccine. Their reasons vary—from worry about long-term effects, through fertility, to inaccurate ideas about microchips and government surveillance.
>
> I find these self-destructive decisions incomprehensible.

There is also the question of free riding. The unvaccinated enjoy the benefits—social freedoms and much reduced risk of covid infection—because the majority of adults, and now adolescents, choose to take the vaccine.

For the first time in my professional life, I am angry with patients who chose not to get vaccinated, and while I do not let it affect my patient care, I think it's affecting me.

Three days later, in the Rapid Response section, Dr. Healy offered the following reply:

We know that the trials were ghostwritten, and even though dead patients went missing, likely preferentially among those taking the vaccine, we know that there was a clear excess of trial volunteers dying on the Pfizer vaccine than on placebo.

The supposed miraculous benefits we have heard about centre on fewer infections. There may have been just the same number of infections with the injections damping symptoms, making the vaccinated more likely to spread the virus and kill vulnerable others. We simply don't know if this is the case.

Is it possible MHRA or FDA would approve a treatment that didn't work? The answer is yes. If they knew it didn't work, would they tolerate articles in prestigious journals claiming it did work? The answer is yes—MHRA and FDA have a track record here they cannot escape.

We are told the real-world evidence shows that it is the unvaccinated who are dying in hospitals. This apparent mismatch with the trial evidence needs to be reconciled. The onus is on those advocating mandates who claim RCTs offer the gold-standard evidence to engage with the issue. CDC and MHRA have also had several-fold more reports of deaths immediately after vaccination in one year from Covid vaccines than from all other vaccines combined over a decade. These too need taking into account.

Although I risk being struck off for mentioning these things, this response is not anonymous.[235]

Two days after that, Canada Prime Minister Justin Trudeau delivered his now-famous screed against covid vaccine skeptics:

> There is still a part of the population that is fiercely against it. The don't believe in science/progress and are often very misogynist and racist.
>
> This leads us as a leader and as a country, to make a choice: Do we tolerate these people?[236]

* * *

By the last day of 2021, the covid pandemic had claimed a reported 774,868 lives in the United States and 5,215,745 world-wide. Also, for the year 2021, the first full year of the vax rollout, VAERS had received 7,996 reports of deaths associated with the covid vaccines—a whopping 108 times as many as for all other vaccine products combined.

And again, let us always keep in mind these post-market reporting systems are thought to capture between one and ten percent of adverse events.

CHAPTER SIX

COVID-19 Cases, Hospitalizations, and Deaths— Can the Official Numbers Be Believed?

The Polymerase Chain Reaction

We have already seen that the coronavirus vaccines were rushed on to the market with unprecedented haste. But, we were told, all this was justified by the unique nature of the threat the pandemic posed to civilization. Night after night newscasters warned us about the mounting toll of covid cases, hospitalizations, and deaths. This seems like a good time to step back and take a look at how reliable those figures are.

The figures for COVID-19 cases, hospitalizations, and deaths are based in a large measure on the quantitative PCR test for viral genetic material. PCR stands for Polymerase Chain Reaction, a process for making a large amount of DNA from a small one. This process was invented by the biochemist Kary Mullis, a feat which earned him the 1993 Nobel Prize in Chemistry.

In the polymerase chain reaction, the DNA of interest is placed in a test tube along with nucleotides and heat-resistant DNA polymerase derived from *Thermus aquaticus*, a bacterium normally found at near-boiling temperatures in hot springs and hydrothermal vents. This mixture is heated to separate the twin strands of the DNA double helix and then cooled. Then the DNA polymerase does its work, synthesizing a complementary strand for each of the single strands of DNA and, lo and behold, you now have two copies of the original DNA double helix. Repeat the cycle of heating and cooling, and now you have four copies. Repeat again and you have eight.

Each cycle of heating and cooling doubles the original amount of DNA. Forty cycles of heating and cooling will increase the initial amount of DNA by a factor of two multiplied by itself forty times, or a little over one trillion, and so a tiny soupçon of DNA can be amplified into a very large amount in a very short period of time.

The number of cycles of heating and cooling needed to produce a measurable amount of DNA is called the cycle threshold (Ct). The smaller the initial amount of DNA, the higher the cycle threshold needed to detect it will be. This is an important point.

Why? Because the fact that a small amount of viral genetic material can be found does not necessarily mean a given patient is infected with the virus, or is capable of transmitting the infection to others. It may simply be indicative of a small amount of viral genetic material that was left over after the body had already conquered the infection, or for that matter was just floating around in the environment at the time the sample was taken. The only way to verify a given patient is infected is to take a sample of that patient's body fluids, use it to inoculate cells in culture dishes, and recover intact virus particle from those cells.

A French study of 183 samples found that those with cycle threshold values between thirteen and seventeen all were capable of producing replication-competent virus. As Ct values exceeded seventeen, infectivity dropped sharply. No samples with Ct values above thirty-three could produce replication-competent virus.[237]

Another more comprehensive study by the same researchers of 3,790 samples corroborated these results, finding that less than three percent of samples with Ct values of thirty-five or greater were infectious.[238]

The CDC and the FDA do not specify a specific cycle threshold for a diagnosis of COVID-19, but an article in the *New York Times* reported that most testing companies set that value at forty cycles—a value guaranteed to ensure false positive results.[239]

Moreover, let us always keep in mind that the companies that perform these tests went from zero to tens of millions of tests per month. How many of these tests were performed by inexperienced, hastily-trained staff—raising the possibility of cross-contamination of samples and therefore more false positive results?

It Gets Awkward

There are other ways by which the official numbers of cases, hospitalizations, and deaths may have been inflated. Official CDC guidelines, drawn up by the Council of State and Territorial Epidemiologists, do not even require PCR or any specific laboratory test for a case of COVID-19 to be added to the official numbers. Two symptoms from a checklist of ten, or one symptom from a checklist of five, is enough. These symptoms (fever, chills, headache, etc.) could be the symptoms of any number of other conditions, but no matter. A simple cough can be enough for a diagnosis of COVID-19 to be rendered—provided that, in the diagnostician's judgement, no other diagnosis is more likely.[240]

In regard to deaths, only five percent of those said to have died from the coronavirus had COVID-19 listed as the sole cause on the death certificate. The remaining ninety-five percent had an average of *four* causes or comorbidities each, including influenza, chronic lower respiratory disease, hypertensive disease, ischemic heart disease, cerebrovascular disease, sepsis, malignant neoplasm, diabetes, obesity—the list goes on and on.[241]

So how to decide whether the coronavirus was actually the cause of a given patient's death or just came along for the ride? The law provides diagnosticians and hospitals with a powerful incentive to classify as many hospitalizations and deaths as possible as due to the coronavirus, by means of the Coronavirus Aid, Relief, and Economic Security (CARES) Act, which provides extra reimbursement for COVID-19 cases.

Scott Jensen, a medical doctor and former state senator in Minnesota, told Fox News:

> Any time health care intersects with dollars, it gets awkward. Right now, if you have a COVID-19 admission to the hospital, you'll get paid thirteen thousand dollars. If that COVID-19 patient goes on a ventilator, you'll get thirty-nine thousand dollars—three times as much. Nobody can tell me, after thirty-five years in the world of medicine, that sometimes those kinds of things impact on what we do.[242]

As if all this were not enough, the Federal Emergency Management Agency offers reimbursements of up to nine thousand dollars for funeral expenses per deceased individual who had COVID-19 listed as the cause on the death certificate.[243]

Public health officials charged with making decisions that impact the life and death of millions of people ought to base their decisions on data that is as accurate and unbiased as possible. That doesn't seem to be what is going on here. There are numerous possible sources of error which could lead to an artificially inflated death toll.

And we haven't even mentioned how the actual death toll was inflated by a governor's decision to place thousands of patients with fulminating illness into nursing homes.

Conspiracy Theories

The same Fox News segment mentioned above contained this take from NIAID Director Anthony Fauci:

> You will always have conspiracy theories when you have very challenging public health crises. They are nothing but distractions.[244]

That may be. But as anyone who has ever dealt with a hospital billing department already knows, when all the mistakes are in their favor, you have to wonder.

Given the systematic over-inflation of covid hospitalizations and deaths, and the systematic denial of covid vaccine harms and deaths, how can all this not lead to an exaggeration of the benefits-to-costs ratio of these products?

Schematic mechanism of PCR

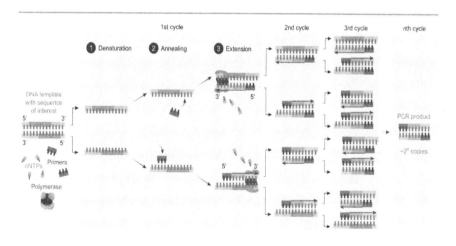

Polymerase chain reaction.[245]

CHAPTER SEVEN

Should People Who Have Recovered from Covid Get the Vax?

CDC and the World Health Organization are united on that point. The WHO admonishes visitors to its website:

> Take whatever vaccine is made available to you first, even if you have already had COVID-19.[246]

The CDC offers similar advice:

> You should get a COVID-19 vaccine even if you already had COVID-19.[247]

The question is, Why? As we have already noted, natural immunity is a fact as well established as the Law of Gravity or the Periodic Table in chemistry. Although it seems not everyone has gotten the message.

On 4 October 2020, amid the darkest days of the covid pandemic, and before the vax had been rolled out, with the world's population chafing under the burden of an ever-shifting mélange of nonsensical restrictions, the American Institute for Economic Research sponsored a conference at Great Barrington, Massachusetts to discuss the official response to the pandemic. At this conference, three eminently credentialed epidemiologists—Sunetra Gupta of Oxford, Martin Kulldorff of Harvard, and Jay Bhattacharya of Stanford—drafted an open letter calling for a more nuanced approach, with targeted protection for vulnerable populations such as the elderly and the infirm, while allowing the young and healthy (who are at miniscule risk for serious complications from the covid) to get on with their lives and in the process acquire immunity to the new pathogen. Known as the Great Barrington Declaration,[248] to many the missive was like a breath of fresh air in an increasingly poisonous debate.

Not everybody saw it that way. The authors found themselves the targets of vitriolic attacks, with NIH Director Francis Collins referring to them as "fringe epidemiologists" in an email to NIAID Director Anthony Fauci, adding "There needs to be a quick and devastating published takedown of its premises."[249] Eight days after the declaration was issued, David Gorski of Science-Based Medicine thundered "COVID-19 deniers follow the path laid down by creationists, HIV/AIDS denialists, and climate deniers."[250] Two days after that, a group of eighty researchers issued a counterproposal published simultaneously in *Lancet* and on a dedicated website, which they christened the "John Snow Memorandum,"[251] after the founding father of epidemiology who discovered the cause of the cholera epidemic in Soho in 1854.[252]

The authors of the memorandum never explained why they felt entitled to borrow moral authority from a man who had been dead for over 150 years and who made his case with argument and evidence, not by smearing and deplatforming his opponents, but never mind that for now. The memorandum contains this curious statement: "There is no evidence for lasting protective immunity to SARS-CoV-2 following natural infection." That may have been true, depending on how one defined "lasting"—when this statement was made, we were less than a year into the pandemic—but since then a plethora of peer-reviewed studies have confirmed what anyone with a working knowledge of the immune system would have predicted—

that natural immunity is robust and durable, with the reduction in the risk of reinfection ranging from eighty percent to one hundred percent.[253]

Moreover, as we have already seen, while some participants who had recovered from the covid were included in the trials, covid infections (as well as serious adverse events, including death) in this population were not counted *as a separate endpoint.* Therefore the effects of vaccination in this population were unknown.

Still, the mainstream medical community continues to endorse the one-size-fits-all approach. Alfred Sommer, Dean Emeritus of the Johns Hopkins Bloomberg School of Public Health, offered this advice in a feature article in the *BMJ*:

> It's a lot easier to put a shot into their arm. To do a PCR test and then process it and then to get the information to them and then to let them think about it—it's a lot easier to just give them the damn vaccine.
>
> I think it's irresponsible from a public health perspective to let people pick and choose what they want to do.[254]

Another argument that has been advanced in favor of vaccinating those recovered from the covid is that natural immunity plus vaccination is superior to natural immunity alone. The same *BMJ* piece quoted Dr. Fauci as endorsing vaccination for the recovered, promising "Your antibodies will go sky-high."[255]

Is that necessarily a good thing? On the one hand, a major study by Israeli researchers showed that, after adjusting for comorbidities, natural immunity plus vaccination significantly reduced the possibility of reinfection by a factor of thirteen times.[256] The incidence of symptomatic COVID-19 and covid-related hospitalizations were reduced as well. (There were no deaths in the study population, in either the experimental group or the control group.) On the other hand, the absolute reduction in risk was tiny—one in eighty-nine for the risk of reinfection—and even less than that for symptomatic covid infections and covid-related hospitalizations.

More importantly, the study had no endpoint for all serious adverse events or all hospitalizations. We have already seen that the damage done by the spike protein is dose-related, and a study of over two thousand patients—mostly health professionals—showed that those who had recovered from the covid had more adverse events and more severe adverse events following vaccination than those who had not.[257]

In the light of all this, Dr. Sommer's admonition to "just give them the damn vaccine" may seem like a blatant repudiation of the very foundation of the doctor-patient relationship, which is that the doctor has a responsibility to do what is best for the patient in front of him, rather than acting as the enforcer of some imagined Greater Good. But it is emblematic of the approach of our Covid Lords, who seemingly insist on treating these complex matters as a one-variable problem.

CHAPTER EIGHT

Should Kids Get the Vax?

We have seen that on 13 May 2021, the CDC recommended extending the Emergency Use Authorization of the Pfizer shot to children between the ages of twelve and fifteen, and on 29 October the EUA was extended to children all the way down to the age of five. The nature of this emergency was not made clear.

Let's take a look at the relevant facts.

Children are at very low risk of complications due to covid infection. In June of 2020, Chinese researchers reported that in a cohort of 2,135 pediatric COVID-19 patients, ninety-four percent had asymptomatic, mild, or moderate cases, and only one had died.[258]

Similar results have been reported in studies from other parts of the world. A white paper released on 11 November 2020 by FAIR Health, the nation's largest private health care claims depository, found that the death rate for children through the age of eighteen diagnosed with COVID-19 was one percent of one percent, or one in ten thousand.[259]

In May of 2021, a team of British researchers reported that between 1 March 2020 through 1 February 2021, out of 137 million children in seven countries (the USA, the UK, Italy, Germany, Spain, France, and South Korea), there had been 231 recorded covid deaths, or one for every six hundred thousand children. These 231 deaths constituted less than one-half of one percent of all childhood mortality.[260]

The next month, clinicians at the Royal Children's Hospital in Melbourne looked at 151 children hospitalized for COVID-19 between 20 March 2020 and 17 March 2021 for whom follow-up data were available for at least three months. Of these 151 children, all had mild or asymptomatic disease and at the most recent review, every single one had returned to his or her baseline health status and all post-acute symptoms had resolved themselves.[261]

The month after that, another team of British researchers analyzed data from children and young people who died of all causes in the UK during the first year of the covid pandemic. There were 3,015 children and young people who died of all causes during that period; of these, sixty-one had tested positive for covid. Analysis of the medical records of these sixty-one patients showed that only twenty-five had died from, rather than with, the covid. The death rate for COVID-19 for children and young people in the first year of the pandemic was one in 500,000. Of the twenty-five children that died from the covid, nineteen had at least one comorbidity, sixteen had multiple comorbidities, and fifteen had a "life-limiting condition."[262]

The same day that study was made available in preprint form, a report by the European Centre for Disease Prevention and Control analyzed data on covid attack rates from the European Surveillance System (TESSY) by age group, sex, and outcome. The study found that children eighteen and under, who made up 16.9 percent the general population, accounted for 15.7 percent of cases. In other words, the rate of infection for children was about the same as that of the general population. However, children accounted for only 1.5 percent of hospitalizations, 0.2 percent of severe hospitalizations, and 0.05 percent of deaths (thirty-seven out of a total of 80,037).[263]

The next month, a study carried out by the American Academy of Pediatrics found that, for the week ending 5 August, in states where data was available, less than two percent of all child COVID-19 cases required hospitalization and the proportion of fatalities ranged from 0.03 percent all the way down to zero.[264]

Moreover, the deliberate disregard for the role of natural immunity had been extended to children, many of whom already have immunity to the covid. A paper published in *Science* on 11 December 2020—before the vax had been rolled out anywhere in the world—found that over sixty percent of *uninfected* children between one and sixteen years of age already had detectable levels of SARS-CoV-2-reactive antibodies in their blood.[265] The following June, before any covid vaccine had been approved for kids anywhere in the world, an Indian study of seven hundred children under eighteen years of age showed that fifty-five percent had antibodies to the coronavirus in their blood.[266]

These figures no doubt underestimate the true level of immunity in this population, as they take into account only humoral immunity, or immunity conferred by the B-cells, and ignore the role played by the other pillar of the body's acquired immune response—T-cell immunity.

Moreover, we have already seen that children seem to be more susceptible than their elders to some of the serious adverse events caused by the vaccine, including myocarditis, which may be the most common and best-documented serious adverse event—and that the risk rises with each subsequent booster

All this would seem to tip the benefits-cost equation away from vaccinating children for the covid.

When I asked Dr. Breggin if kids should get the vax, he did not hesitate before replying:

> The vaccine is of no use to children because they don't get very sick from it. They either have no symptoms or symptoms of a cold. The experts agree that the rate of serious infection in children is zero. There have been one or two or a few reported cases of very ill children dying who also had covid, but they're

so rare and difficult to evaluate that the rate is considered zero for deaths in children.

On the other hand, children are particularly prone to cardiac problems, including myocarditis, and that is a very dangerous disorder.

It would be better to hold COVID-19 parties for children where they got infected from each other than to isolate them, because they will develop a very excellent immunity if they get it as children. This will protect them better than any known vaccine, and will contribute more to the benefit of society by creating a generation of children who will have herd immunity.

With the vaccines, you will kill a certain number of children. It's not clear yet how many. You will sterilize a significant number of them. It could be as high as thirty percent. The data is not in yet. There's an infinite number of reasons not to vaccinate the children and no harm from avoiding vaccinating them.

This is a no brainer.

Some might argue that children should be vaxxed anyway, to protect their elders. Some early reports that children are not a source of viral transmission turned out, unfortunately, to be overly optimistic. There are cases of children transmitting the virus to other children and to adults. But that begs the question of whether the shot stops transmission—and we have already seen the data indicates it does not.

Moreover, children have already borne a disproportionate share of the burden of pandemic restrictions on their little shoulders, and if vaxxing kids does not confer a net benefit to them, it should not be considered. Anyone who says otherwise is saying, in effect, that he is willing to use children as human shields. Aren't we better than that?

CHAPTER NINE

The Pfizer Data Dump Commences

January–February 2022

A One-in-Two-Hundred-Year Catastrophe

On the first day of the new year, the news website Center Square reported that Scott Davison, CEO of the Indianapolis-based insurance company OneAmerica, had reported that the death rate for working-age adults had risen by a staggering forty percent from pre-pandemic levels.[267] Davison told the reporter:

> We're seeing, right now, the highest death rates we have seen in the history of this business—not just at OneAmerica. The data is consistent across every player in that business.
>
> Just to give you an idea of how bad that is, a three-sigma or a one-in-200-year catastrophe would be 10% increase over pre-pandemic. So 40% is just unheard of.

Davison added that most claims were not for deaths recorded as due to COVID-19. He did not offer an explanation as to what was causing the excess mortality.

The figure of a forty percent increase in excess deaths was widely circulated on social media, with many posters concluding that the vax was the cause. The self-styled "fact-checkers" swung into play, with both the Associated Press[268] and PolitiFact[269] rating the story "false" and claiming that covid deaths were in fact being undercounted.

The fact-checkers had a point when they asserted that no one had proven that the increase in deaths was caused by the vax. But they provided no evidence that covid deaths were being undercounted, and in fact they went preposterously beyond the available evidence when they flatly stated the excess deaths had not been caused by the shot, without explaining how they could know this.

The fact-checkers also neglected to mention that, like CNN, PolitiFact is funded by the Bill and Melinda Gates Foundation.[270]

Ghoulish, but Necessary

On 4 January, in an interview with *Le Parisien*, French President Emmanuel Macron proclaimed:

> Eh bien là, les non-vaccinés, j'ai très envie de les emmerder.[271]

The English-language media dutifully (and demurely) translated *emmerder* as "to piss off," but that is not the meaning of the word.

In plain English: the president of a major nation, speaking on the record in an interview with a major media outlet, said he wanted to shit on the unvaccinated.

Six days after that, a headline in the *Los Angeles Times* proclaimed "Mocking Anti-Vaxxers' Covid Deaths Is Ghoulish, Yes,—But May Be Necessary."[272] The very next day, an essay in the *Washington Post* proclaimed "Macron is Right: It's Time to Make Life a Living Hell for Anti-Vaxxers."[273]

Four days later, a headline in the *Toronto Star* confronted readers with this poignant question:

The Unvaccinated Cherish Their Freedom to Harm Others.
How Can We Ever Forgive Them?[274]

One week after that, the Canadian Broadcasting Corporation News ran a story titled "Public Outrage over the Unvaccinated is Driving a Crisis in Bioethics," which stated:

> Vaccinated majorities in wealthy western countries are growing increasingly impatient with a science-denying minority being blamed for prolonging the pandemic and stretching critical care resources to the breaking point.[275]

The piece never actually came out and *said* the unvaccinated should be denied life-saving health care (and in fact it quoted two doctors as well as the editor of the journal *Bioethics* who came out against the idea) but the overall intention clearly seemed to be to leave the proposal on the table, as a titillating possibility. The article also never examined the role of media outlets such as the Canadian Broadcasting Corporation in whipping up "public outrage over the unvaccinated."

Three days later, after UK Prime Minister Boris Johnson lifted most covid restrictions, the *Mirror* published a diatribe by columnist Polly Hudson. Some selections follow:

> Get jabbed, or else. It sounds harsh, and it is—but the time has come where it's essential.
>
> The best thing we can do is protect ourselves is get vaccinated and boosted. Then your chances of catching Covid are reduced, but even if you do, you're much less likely to be seriously ill, or—crucially for society—to spread it to others.
>
> The militant, rabid anti-vaxxers will never be persuaded, so they need to be forced.
>
> No excuses. Too many people who happily put meals containing who-knows-what chemicals into their bodies, or

those who ingest recreational drugs cut with let's-not-even-go-there have said they won't have the jab because they don't know what's in it.

Unless you're a food chemist or a drug dealer, nobody knows what's in anything! The vaccine has been tested and proven. Get jabbed or else.

The unvaccinated must become social pariahs.

They shouldn't be allowed into indoor communal spaces like restaurants, cinemas, shops, gigs, and—yup, the most bitter of all blows—pubs.

Why should those of us who are jabbed and boosted have to risk breathing in their maskless air?[276]

Robust Protection

Meanwhile, a study by researchers in Qatar published on 6 January reported that prior infection with COVID-19 resulted in a sixty percent reduction in the likelihood of reinfection with the new Omicron strain.[277] The protection against Omicron afforded by prior immunity was significantly less than the degree of protection against earlier strains, but far greater than the protection offered by vaccination. Moreover, out of 412 cases of reinfection, there were only two cases of severe covid and no deaths.

The study authors concluded "Prior-infection protection against hospitalization or death at reinfection appears robust, regardless of variant."

The Public Has a Right

The same day the Qatari study appeared in preprint form, the United States Northern District Court of Texas ordered the FDA to begin releasing the Pfizer trial data, beginning with twelve thousand pages no later than 31 January and continuing at a rate of fifty-five thousand pages per month, rather than the puny five hundred pages the agency had offered.

Thirteen days later, in a piece in the *BMJ*, Dr. Doshi and two colleagues lauded the release but claimed it did not go far enough.[278] They pointed out that the court order pertained only to the Pfizer shot, not the Moderna vax nor any of the other covid vaccine products available.

The authors concluded:

> Data must be made available when the trial results are announced, published, or used to justify government regulatory decisions. There is no place for wholesale exemptions from good practice during a pandemic. The public has paid for covid-19 vaccines through vast public funding of research, and it is the public that has taken on the benefits and harms that accompany vaccination. The public, therefore, has a right and entitlement to those data, as well as to the interrogation of those data by experts.
>
> The purpose of regulators is not to dance to the tune of rich global corporations and enrich them further; it is to protect the health of their populations. We need complete data transparency for all studies, and we need it now.

Yet again all of these words of caution fell upon deaf ears.

That same day, Dr. Healy published a lengthy piece in his RxISK blog titled "The Evidence That Counts for FDA,"[279] in which he detailed the myriad problems with industry-sponsored trials, ending with this summary:

1) Clinicians do not have access to clinical trial data on medicines or vaccines.

2) Close to all of the medical literature reporting trial results for on-patent drugs and vaccines is ghostwritten, hyping the benefits and hiding the harms.

3) Clinical trials of these treatments that are negative on their primary or their most common outcomes are often published in prestigious journals as positive.

4) Clinical trials have their harms airbrushed out of ghost-written publications.

5) Regulators (FDA, Health Canada, MHRA, EMA) do not get to see the full trial data.

6) Regulators approve treatments as working even when more people die on active treatment than on placebo.

7) Regulators approve medicines on the basis of negative studies and agree not to let the wider world know about this.

8) Regulators say nothing when companies publish negative studies as positive and make adverse effects of treatment, including death, vanish.

9) For many trials there are more deaths on active treatment than on placebo, but this does not lead regulators to warn about hazards as to do so would in their stated view deter people from seeking a benefit (even when the benefit is better characterized as a commercial benefit to a company rather than a benefit to the individual in terms of a life saved or a restoration of function).

The entire document was sent to:

- Joe Biden
- The British Medical Association
- Sajid Javid, Secretary of State for Health and Social Care in the United Kingdom
- Eluned Morgan, Minister for Health in Wales
- Robin Swann, Minister for Health in Northern Ireland

- The MHRA

- NICE

- Daniel Sokol, a lawyer with an interest in ethical issues who has written in favor of mandates

- Jeff King, another lawyer who has written in favor of mandates

- The Canadian Health Minister

- The Chief Public Health Officer for Ontario

- The Ontario Human Rights Commission

- The College of Physicians and Surgeons of Ontario (CPSO)

- The President of McMaster University

- The Dean of Medicine at McMaster University

Not one of these eminently credentialed experts or prestigious organizations disputed any of his points.

In a follow-up post one week later, Dr. Healy wrote:

> In the case of vaccines, it is very clear that healthy people, many of them enthusiastically pro-vaccine, as well as others driven by fear of the virus or losing a job, are being killed and seriously injured by these mRNA agents. When injured they meet medical systems and personnel who ridicule them and tell them their problems are in their mind or the pain in their chest is a sign that the vaccine is working.
>
> Doctors and nurses have lost jobs for linking injuries and vaccines. This inhibits others from doing so and blocks the possibility of early diagnoses that might encourage research on these injuries and lead to treatments that might minimize disability and prevent deaths.
>
> It now appears to be the norm for doctors facing a patient with thrombosis, myocarditis, peripheral neuropathy or other

problems following a first dose of a Covid vaccine to refuse to endorse an application for a medical exemption from the second dose. In this case, the doctor is de facto denying a causal link to treatment. It's a bizarre abrogation of the role of a physician.

If a doctor writes a letter supporting an exemption, this will ordinarily be turned down by another person in the system, commonly working in public health, who has never met and will never meet the injured person and will almost certainly have less medical expertise in managing that injury than the person supporting the exemption.

Over the past three decades, the encroachment of a fake literature paraded as gold standard evidence has produced soft mandates that have eroded the likelihood that patients will get justice in clinical settings for injuries stemming from SSRIs, statins for cholesterol, bisphosphonates for osteo-porosis, other drugs used to manage risks, and the mRNA agents now designated as vaccines.

The addition of hard mandates for these mRNA agents can only make things worse.

The argument outlined here is not based on the rights of individuals to bodily autonomy. It speaks to the wider rights of all of us to the benefits that stem from all of us co-op-erating in accordance with the jointly held values that are embodied in what we call science and justice.[280]

Ground Zero

The erosion of freedom, exacerbated by vaccine mandates, should concern us all.

Early in the pandemic, our knowledge was minimal. But because of what we learned from Italy and the Princess Cruise ship, it was obvious that covid was a disease that targeted the old and those with certain comorbidities. Instead of using that information, public health officials pursued a one-size-fits-all response that relied heavily on a state of fear to ensure compliance.

They also kept moving the goalposts.

And as goalposts were moving, different viewpoints were being crushed.

So said Senator Ron Johnson at the panel discussion "COVID-19: A Second Opinion" held at the Russell Senate Office Building in Washington, DC on Monday, 24 January 2022.

The audience comprised another motley assortment of free-lance journalists, bloggers, patient advocates, and their families, while the panel featured some of the nation's top clinicians and scientists who have dissented from the mainstream narrative regarding the pandemic. But again, almost as notable was the list of dignitaries who were invited but declined to attend, including CDC Director Rochelle Walensky, Acting FDA Commissioner Janet Woodcock, former NIH Director Francis Collins, former FDA Director Scott Gottlieb (who, as we have noted, now serves on the board of Pfizer), and—last but not least—NIAID Director and Chief Medical Advisor to the President of the United States, Anthony Fauci.

Again, also conspicuous by their absence were any representatives of the legacy media.

The discussion had been scheduled to run from 9:00 AM to 12:00 Noon but in fact continued long after that and included a wide range of topics, including covid vaccines, vaccine mandates, lockdowns, masks, and the suppression of safe and effective early-stage treatment for

COVID-19—the *sine qua non* of the Emergency Use Authorization for the covid vaccines.

Peter McCullough, former Vice Chief of Internal Medicine at Baylor University Medical Center, gave the opening statement. He pointed out that all the doctors at the round table use vaccines in their practice, but cautioned "Never have we widely applied vaccination in the middle of a pandemic."

David Wiseman, Internal Medicine Specialist at MedStar Union Memorial Hospital, compared repeated booster shots to a Whack-A-Mole game, describing the strategy as "Neither sustainable nor smart," adding ominously "The wounds of vaccine divisiveness will take decades to heal."

Then Aaron Kheriaty addressed the panel. Until recently, Dr. Kheriaty had been Professor of Psychiatry at the University of California Irvine School of Medicine and Director of the Medical Ethics Program at UCI Health, but he was fired from his position after questioning the constitutionality of vaccine mandates.

> I want to talk about medical ethics. Because I'm concerned that many of our pandemic policies have ignored foundational principles of medical ethics. We effectively abandoned patients that were suffering from other conditions and had other medical needs.
>
> The disastrous fruits of this myopia include an unprecedented forty percent increase in all-cause mortality among working-age adults over the last year. Most of which—two third to three quarters, depending on the state—was not related to covid. Actuaries tell us that a ten percent rise in all-cause mortality is a once-in-two-hundred-year disaster. This was a forty percent rise.

Dr. Kheriaty decried the absurdity of vaxxing those who had already recovered from the covid: "There is not a single report of a person recovering and then transmitting the virus."

He went on to state that it was currently impossible to obtain a vaccine exemption in the state of California, even for patients who had known life-threatening complications from the vax.

"There is no clearer contraindication to a medicine than already having been harmed by that medicine," he told the panel, adding angrily "A four-year-old could have figured that one out."

Brianne Dressen was there as well. Speaking of the vaccine-injured, she had this to say:

> Eighty percent of us are diagnosed with anxiety initially, and then months down the road that's when we get appropriate diagnoses. And that's when we actually are able to find doctors that are willing to go against the directive—because like these physicians were discussing, their licenses have been threatened—and because their licenses have been threatened, we cannot get medical care. They are afraid to treat us.
>
> We have had patients who are severely injured and are dying who cannot get in the door to get seen by physicians because physicians are afraid of the word "covid vaccine." So instead what they are doing is they've made us—like Kyle Warner and myself and our membership of over twelve thousand covid-vaccine-injured—we are Ground Zero to take care of the covid-vaccine-injured, when we have highly qualified practitioners across the globe that have been silenced and threatened if they even so much as see us for what's going on.

Dropping a Bombshell

Long after the discussion had been scheduled to end, trial lawyer Tom Renz took the stand. Renz, a big blocky man with strong features and a booming voice, proceeded to drop a bombshell.

The attorney informed the members he was currently representing three Department of Defense physicians: Lieutenant Colonel Theresa Long, Lt. Col. Peter Chambers, and Dr. Samuel Sigoloff, who had come forward with some potentially explosive allegations. The three docs claimed the rate of serious adverse events among military personnel skyrocketed after the introduction of the COVID-19 vaccine, in comparison to the years 2016-2020. These serious adverse events included:

- A 302% increase in tachycardia
- A 369% increase in testicular cancer
- A 437% increase in ovarian dysfunction
- A 452% increase in migraines
- A 468% increase in pulmonary embolism
- A 472% increase in female infertility
- A 474% increase in neoplasms of the thyroid and other endocrine glands
- A 487% increase in demyelinating
- A 487% increase in breast cancer
- A 551% increase in Guillain-Barré syndrome
- A 624% increase in cancers of the digestive system
- A 680% increase in multiple sclerosis
- A 900% increase in esophageal cancer
- A 1048% increase in diseases of the nervous system

• And a whopping 2200% increase in hypertension

The reader will note that all of these events can be linked to the toxic spike protein.

Renz provided data downloaded by unnamed DoD whistleblowers from the Defense Medical Epidemiology Database (DMED) personnel validating all this.

"Our own soldiers are being experimented on and killed," Renz told the panel.

After the hearing was concluded, Senator Johnson fired off a letter to the Department of Defense demanding an explanation. On 1 February, the DoD contacted the website Lead Stories and confirmed all of Renz's claims, but they attributed the apparent rise in serious adverse events to a "technical glitch" which caused serious adverse events to be under-reported for the years 2016-2020, and they claimed to have taken DMED offline while they took steps to "identify and correct the root-cause of their data corruption."[281] The Lead Stories Piece did not explain why this "glitch" went unnoticed for five years, nor why it mysteriously corrected itself just in time for the vax rollout.

Shamefully, this story has been completely ignored by the legacy media.

Four days after the meeting of the expert panel, I published an account of the event on my blog at Medium. Within hours, my Medium account was canceled.

It Doesn't Make Sense

On the first day of February, Pfizer requested the FDA authorize for emergency use the two-dose regimen of Comirnaty for children below five years of age, using a three-microgram dose of spike protein mRNA, rather than the standard ten micrograms for patients between the ages of five and eleven, and thirty for those aged twelve and older. In a press release, the company noted that the trial that formed the basis for this request was designed to evaluate the safety, tolerability, and immunogenicity of the shot, but did not even try to claim the data showed their product reduced the frequency of covid infection of any intensity, let alone severe infection, deaths, hospitalizations, intubations, transmission, or any other clinically relevant outcome.[282]

The primary endpoint for the trial was antibody levels, and even this low bar proved too difficult to surmount. The company's own data showed the vax failed to produce a robust immune response in two-to-four-year-olds. Only in tots between the ages of six months and two years did the shot produce the hoped-for levels of antibodies, and in fact the request for emergency use authorization came at the prompting of the FDA.[283]

The question is, Why? The FDA wanted to give parents a head start on vaccinating their preschool-age children with the first two doses so they would be ready for the third dose by the time that was approved.[284]

Pfizer CEO Albert Bourla proclaimed:

> Ultimately, we believe that three doses of the vaccine will be needed for children 6 months through 4 years of age to achieve high levels of protection against current and potential future variants. If two doses are authorized, parents will have the opportunity to begin a COVID-19 vaccination series for their children while awaiting potential authorization of a third dose.

FDA officials noted that the trial data (which were still unpublished) had not demonstrated the two-dose regimen had caused the little ones any harm.[285] But that's setting the bar pretty low. Isn't the whole point of giving the shot to children to make them *better*?

The sheer blinding fatuity of giving toddlers two doses of a vaccine which had not been shown to produce any clinical benefits, in order to prepare them for the third dose still being trialed, was lost on some. Yvonne Maldonado, Professor of Clinical Pediatric Infectious Disease at Stanford, told the *New York Times* "There's almost no conceivable hypothesis where a third dose would be worse"[286]—ignoring the possibility of myocarditis, along with any other toxic effects of the spike protein which might be dose-dependent.

This optimism was not shared by all. Paul Offit, Director of Vaccine Education at Philadelphia Children's Hospital and a member of the FDA Advisory Panel, told a reporter "It doesn't make sense we would approve a two-dose vaccine on the assumption that the third dose would make up for the deficiency of the two doses."[287]

The next day, the Northern District Court of Texas order regarding the Pfizer documents was modified as follows:

- 10,000 pages apiece due on or before 1 March and on 1 April

- 80,000 pages apiece due on or before 2 May, 1 June, and 1 July

- 70,000 pages due on or before 1 August

- 55,000 pages apiece due on the first business day of the month thereafter until the release of the documents is completed

The day after that, a paper in *Frontiers in Public Health* assessed adverse reactions to both the covid vaccines and the influenza vaccine that had been reported to both VAERS and to the European Database of Suspected Adverse Drug Reactions (EudraVigilance) between December 2020 (when the covid vax was rolled out) through October 2021.[288] The total number of people exposed to the covid vax was 451 million, as opposed to 437 million for the influenza shot. The researchers calculated the relative risk of serious adverse events associated with the covid shot as opposed to the flu shot, and found the covid shot was associated with an increased risk for a number of adverse events, including allergic reactions, arrhythmia, general cardiovascular events, coagulation, hemorrhages, gastrointestinal effects, ocular effects, effects on the sex organs, and thrombosis.

The reader will note that all of these events can be linked to the toxic spike protein.

The most interesting part of the paper was Table 1, which shows the relative risk of hospitalizations, life-threatening reactions, and deaths per one hundred thousand patients for the covid shot, as compared to the flu shot. The results were nothing short of astonishing.

Event	EudraVigilance	VAERS
Hospitalizations	46	190
Life-Threatening Reactions	43	197
Deaths	56	345

In plain English: in comparison to the flu shot, the number of deaths reported to VAERS in association with the covid shot, per hundred thousand doses, was elevated by a staggering three hundred and forty-five times.

Eight days later, the CDC announced that the efficacy of the COVID-19 booster shot declined sharply after four months, and suggested another booster might be necessary.[289] That next day, the FDA announced it would delay emergency use authorization of the Pfizer vax for children under the age of five until results from the three-dose series were in. The decision was made after Pfizer reported the two-dose series was "not sufficiently effective" in preventing symptomatic infection in tots as the Omicron variant surged.[290]

Two days after that, the *Epoch Times* reported that Brook Jackson was going ahead with her lawsuit she had filed against Pfizer and Ventavia under the False Claims Act, despite the US government refusing to assist her. Government lawyers declined to give an explanation, and the FDA did not respond to a request for comment.[291]

That same day, New York City fired over a thousand municipal workers for refusing the covid shots.[292] Although this number represented less than one percent of the city's work force, it was believed to have been the single largest mass firing in the country's history in response to a vaccine mandate.[293]

The day after that, Dr. Healy announced the inauguration of a new Cause and Effect forum on his personal blog for case histories of patients harmed by covid vaccines,[294] beginning with this opening salvo:

> Any previous vaccine program that had a fraction of the numbers of reports to the Vaccine Adverse Events Reporting System (VAERS), run by the US Centers for Disease Control (CDC), as the Covid vaccines have had would have been suspended a month or two into the vaccine roll-out. But not this one. The reports of harms get written off as anecdotes. "Anyone can report to the VAERS System, you know, are you sure these aren't just coming off bots?"

Dr. Healy explained that this forum had its genesis at the expert panel meeting convened by Senator Ron Johnson the previous November:

> There is no question in my mind that the 10 people talking about their injuries at this meeting had been injured in just the way they claimed. Maybe they were the only 10 people in the world who had ever been injured by the vaccines (all 4 of the major vaccines) but the idea that these injuries were non-existent, co-incidental, or all in the minds of these 10 was just wrong.

In a follow-up post, Dr. Healy presented the first of ten case histories, that of Brianne Dressen, and threw down the gauntlet to his professional colleagues:

The publication of these cases challenges anyone who thinks the vaccines cannot cause a problem to accept that in these instances they have caused problems. If you don't think they have caused a problem, there is an invitation to interview the people here, in this case Bri, and see if you can spot a more plausible way to explain what has happened.

To take up this challenge, you must be prepared to have your name and your credentials to undertake an assessment made public along with a recording of your examination and report. Names and running the experiment in front of people are key elements of the scientific process.[295]

Fanning the Flames

The same day Dr. Healy announced the inauguration of his Cause and Effect Forum, hate speech against covid vaccine skeptics reached what was perhaps its all-time extreme during a debate in the Canadian House of Commons.[296] Conservative MP Melissa Lantsman accused Prime Minister Justin Trudeau of "fanning the flames of an unjustified national emergency," adding "When did the Prime Minster lose his way?"

This was the Prime Minister's reply:

> Conservative party members can stand with people who wave swastikas. They can stand with people who wave the Confederate flag.
>
> We will choose to stand with Canadians who deserve to be able to get to their jobs, to be able to get their lives back.

Lantsman, the descendant of Holocaust survivors, replied:

> I am a strong Jewish woman. I have never been made to feel less, except for today, when the Prime Minister accused me of

standing with swastikas. I would like an apology, and I think he owes an apology to all members of the House.

In response to her demand for an apology, MP Lantsman was told "The Prime Minister has left the House."[297]

Data Corruption

The same day Prime Minister Trudeau put all of his wit on display in the House of Parliament, Lt. Col. Theresa Long was testifying on behalf of two Uniformed Services officers (one Navy, one in the Marine Corps) who had filed suit after being denied a religious exemption from covid vaccine mandates.[298] The DoD lawyers produced an unsigned document stating:

> In January of 2022, Department Officials found that data in DMED covering the years 2016-2020 had been corrupted during an August 2021 server migration.

The judge admonished the DoD for failing to produce any expert witness to back up this claim, but never mind that for now. Why hadn't the DoD said anything about a server migration when they contacted Lead Stories (in lieu of responding directly to Senator Johnson's query) two weeks earlier?

A Disturbing Possibility

Meanwhile, the evidence for the lack of long-term effectiveness of the covid vaccines against the Omicron variant continued to mount. A report that had been published the previous month by the UK Health Security Agency reviewed a number of studies and concluded that the efficacy of the covid vaccine against the new Omicron variant dropped to somewhere between ten percent and zero just six months after two doses. A third dose was said to bring the efficacy back up to somewhere between forty and fifty percent (just barely at or even below the FDA's minimum standard of effectiveness) between four and six months, but there were "insufficient data" to draw any conclusions for the vaccine's efficacy after that. The researchers rated the evidence as "high confidence," meaning the evidence came from multiple studies and was consistent and comprehensive.[299]

Despite this, no one seemed interested in re-considering the wisdom of trying to vaccinate our way out of the pandemic, nor the possible cumulative effects of repeated inundations of the toxic spike protein, with the authors of one of the aforementioned studies instead calling out for "a massive rollout of vaccinations and booster vaccinations."[300]

A report by the Health Advisory and Recovery Team (HART) Group released 17 February suggested an explanation for the lack of long-term effectiveness of the covid vaccines.[301] In a previous report, they had pointed out that rate of infections following each successive wave of the pandemic followed a Gompertz curve, characterized by a sharp increase followed by a constant rate of slowing, with only about five to fifteen percent of the population being infected by any given strain of the virus. This suggests that only a small portion of the population is susceptible to any given strain, and once the virus sweeps through that portion (perhaps aided by increasing rates of infection in the first two weeks after vaccination), the rate of infection will decline until the next variant is introduced.[302]

The authors pointed out that if waning immunity was due to some property of the vax itself, we would expect to see the same time to waning immunity in every country. In fact, the data showed the time to "waning immunity" varied wildly from country to country, but that it correlated almost perfectly with the arrival of each new variant.[303]

This was an astounding revelation. Hundreds of millions of people had been induced to get this experimental gene therapy with no long-term safety data shot into their bodies. The idea that the effectiveness of the shot could disappear so quickly was disturbing enough, but the HART Group was suggesting an even more disturbing possibility—that "waning immunity" was an illusion concealing the fact that the vax never was effective in the first place.

Three days later the *New York Times* revealed that the CDC had suppressed its own data on the lack of effectiveness of boosters in adults aged eighteen through forty-nine. The article quoted CDC spokesperson Kristen Nordlund who offered this explanation for not releasing the data it had collected at taxpayer expense:

> Because basically, at the end of the day, it's not yet ready for prime time.[304]

She also noted that releasing information on the lack of effectiveness of booster shots might be used to discourage people from getting those shots.

This was an astonishing admission. The CDC was telling us, in effect, that its own data contradicted its policies and that, rather than change the policies, it chose to keep those data hidden.

Two days after that *Fierce Healthcare* reported that thousands of hospital employees nationwide had been fired from their jobs for refusing the vax.[305] This was more than a bit ironic, given that one of the reasons commonly given for forcing people to get the shot was to avoid strain on the hospital system.

A Stroke of Bad Luck

Late in the morning of Saturday 26 February I put the finishing touches on my third book, which was about the toxic effects of ADHD drugs. It felt good finally to begin the process of getting this off my plate so I could devote more time to new projects. Even though I had included a chapter titled "ADHD in the Time of Covid," anything that happened before December of 2019 was starting to feel like ancient history.

Dr. Healy had given me the name of a woman who had generously agreed to provide free copy-editing services, and so I emailed her, and while I was waiting for her to reply I decided to go for a walk. As I was trudging along Deepdene Road, a path I had trodden hundreds of times before, my right arm suddenly felt cold and heavy and stiff, as if it had been pumped up with ice water. I tried shaking it off, and I resolved to finish my walk, but then my right foot began slipping out from under me with every step I took. Nothing like this had ever happened to me before, so I pulled out my cell phone and called my wife.

"Come and get me right now," I told her.

"What is wrong?" she asked.

"Come and get me RIGHT NOW!"

It occurred to me that less than thirty days had elapsed since I'd had my booster shot.

Medically, it had made no sense for me to get the vax. I'd already had the covid, and I'd recovered fully in just a few days, without taking any medicine at all. But I'd gotten the shot to protect my health—because if I hadn't, I would have been unemployed and broke and homeless, and that would have been hazardous to my health.

Now at the age of sixty, after twenty-nine years of teaching without missing a single day of work due to illness, I was suffering from an ischemic stroke.

I staggered back to the Starbucks at the corner of Deepdene Road and Roland Avenue and sat down at one of their outdoor tables, and my wife arrived and drove me to the hospital where she worked, and they gave me the shot of their miracle clot-busting drug, and within three hours I was sitting up in bed and eating a late lunch and feeling good as new.

The next day I asked the neurologist point-blank "Do you think the shot caused this?" His answer almost knocked me off my feet:

> Well, we're now seeing eighteen-year-olds coming in with strokes, and in those cases it's pretty obvious what's causing it, but for someone your age it's not so clear-cut.

Who could argue with that?

They kept me in hospital for two days and ran all kinds of tests on me, as if they were desperate to find something to blame it on besides the shot. They didn't find anything. They even had me wear a heart monitor for the next thirty days. That study failed to turn up anything, either.

What else can I tell you? The nurses were all friendly and welcoming, the docs were all polished and professional and at the same time oozing empathy, the food was fresh, plentiful, and attractively presented on china plates, with both of my evening meals coming garnished with an atorvastatin tablet prominently displayed on the tray, as if it were an after-dinner mint—literally handing them out like candy. (I didn't take the thing.)

And, unfortunately, they had placed me on their low-sodium diet, so no added salt.

Although I could get all the packets of sugar I wanted.

The bill for two days amounted to $9,435—although my wife's insurance policy paid all but fifteen bucks. I sometimes wonder why shepherding old people to their deaths is a job that merits health insurance coverage, but teaching the next generation of young people is not. But that's a topic for another book.

As of 15 May 2022, the date of my writing this, there had been 418 reports of ischemic stroke associated with the covid vaccines processed by the VAERS database—eleven times as many as for all other vaccines combined since the reporting system was initiated.

After my release Dr. Healy kindly offered to take a look at my medical records. After reviewing them he emailed me:

> I'd imagine your BP was a little up in the ER but the diastolic looked great
>
> Hard to see what you sd do except not research it all too much and keep walking
>
> D

Indeed. Compared to a lot of people, I got off lightly. And I have no doubt that during my time in hospital I received the very best care modern medicine has to offer. Although I would have greatly preferred not to have needed it in the first place.

CHAPTER TEN

The Pfizer Data Dump Continues

March–May 2022

Missing Context

On Tuesday 1 March, the first trove of Pfizer documents was released, as promised. Of mild interest was the "Prescription Drug User Fee Coversheet" which documented a payment of $2,875,822.00 to the FDA. Of more interest was a thirty-eight-page document titled "Cumulative Analysis of Post-Authorization Adverse Event Reports of PF-07302048 (BNT162B2) Received Through 28 February 2021." In the first less than three months after the vax was rolled out, the company received 42,086 adverse events reports including 1,223 deaths. The total number of vaccine doses administered during this time had been redacted for "business reasons."

The figure of 1,223 reported deaths was widely distributed on social media, and again the self-styled "fact checkers" swung into play. Reuters rated the story as "Missing context,"[306] *Newsweek* as "Misleading,"[307] and *USA Today* as "False."[308]

The fact checkers had a point when they stated that reporting to post-marketing surveillance systems is not proof of causality. However, they neglected to mention that such systems generally are assumed to capture between one and ten percent of all adverse events (some estimates are even less than one percent, but no one really knows). They also neglected to mention that (as we have already seen) the swine flu vaccine was pulled off the market in 1976 after just five hundred cases of Guillain-Barré Syndrome and twenty-five deaths. So the fact checkers were themselves "missing context."

Indeed, the *USA Today* piece went far beyond missing context. This was their opening salvo:

> As health care officials continue to urge Americans to get vaccinated and the coronavirus has led to more than 1 million deaths in the U.S., some online posts falsely claim the Pfizer COVID-19 vaccine makes people sick and kills them.

The author seemed to be saying that *any* claims of adverse events or deaths due to the vaccine are false. Not even Pfizer was claiming that. And, as we have already seen, the claim of one million deaths due to the coronavirus is also suspect—to say the least. Has *USA Today* crossed over the line from "Missing context" to out-and-out falsehoods?

We Are Not Willing to Engage in This Discussion

On 4 March, Senator Johnson and nine of his Republican colleagues dispatched a message to all of their colleagues in the Senate, declaring they would not consent to the passage of any continuing resolution or omnibus bill that funded covid vaccine mandates.

Three days after that, the senator issued a letter to Unissant, the corporation responsible for managing the Defense Medical Epidemiology Database (DMED). This database had been the object of shocking allegations made by attorney Tom Renz in the course of the panel discussion held at the Senate Office Building on 24 January.

A member of Senator Johnson's staff had emailed the company the previous week. A Unissant employee responded "We are not in a position nor are we willing to engage in this discussion."

In his latest missive, Senator Johnson requested that Unissant:

- Explain the company's contractual obligations to the DoD
- List all other instances of "data corruption" that have occurred in the database
- Provide all documents and communications between Unissant and the DoD referring or relating to DMED from 1 August 2021 to the present
- Preserve all records referring, relating, or reported to DMED

Moonshot

Monday 8 March saw the publication of Albert Bourla's autobiographical *Moonshot*,[309] his version of the events leading up to and following of the deployment of the Pfizer vax. The book was a carefully crafted masterpiece of public relations, extolling the brilliance and dedication of his employees and even leavening the tale with a dash of humility, expressing contrition for the times when, in the heat of the moment, Dr. Bourla had let his emotions get the better of him and lashed out at his faithful followers. All due to his deep and abiding concern for the rest of us, of course.

Dr. Bourla also notes that both of his parents are Holocaust survivors and goes on to mention that his mother, as a young teenage girl, had been confined to the Jewish ghetto in Thessaloniki and was forced to wear a yellow star every time she ventured outside its confines—in effect turning her into an alien in her own country.

The irony of all this seems to have been lost on Dr. Bourla.

An All-Time High

On 18 March, the *Guardian* reported that covid cases were resurging across the UK, with the number of cases in those over seventy years of age reaching an all-time high[310]—despite that fact that nearly one hundred percent of people in that age group had received at least one vaccine dose.[311]

Was this due to original antigenic sin (which the experts had warned us about before the vax rollout), antibody-dependent enhancement (which the experts had also warned about), or some combination of the two? Nobody really knew—but why this was happening was nowhere near as important as that it was happening.

This was an astonishing finding. But rather than admit the obvious— that the vax wasn't working as intended—the article quoted a distinguished expert from Oxford University who called for more boosters.

Revisions

On 22 March, Mathew Crawford, a fellow at the Institute for Advanced Cultural Studies at the University of Virginia, published a Substack post about the safety signals in DMED. Crawford had examined the data closely, and compared the data with that found in the *Medical Surveillance Monthly Reports*, available at health.mil.[312]

Every May, the *MSMR* publishes summary data on ambulatory and hospital visits recorded in DMED for three staggered previous years—for example, in May 2021 they published data for the years 2016, 2018, and 2020. In May 2019 they published data for the years 2014, 2016, and 2018. And so forth.

Crawford compared data from the 2019 *MSMR* report with that from the 2021 report, and also from DMED query data dated 14 February 2022. In 2021 and 2022, the reported number of ambulatory visits for many categories of adverse events 2016 and 2018 was revised upwards compared to what was reported in 2019.

What's more, these upward revisions were not randomly distributed. Events believed to be associated with the covid vax underwent more drastic increases than those not. For example, while all reports of ambulatory events associated with the circulatory system rose by 21.2%, reports of acute myocarditis rose by 48.3%, acute pericarditis 99.5%, and hypertensive disease a staggering 2,381.3%.

Crawford told readers:

> Given the observation of the large revisions, it is not simply unprecedented, but shocking to see neither asterisk (*) nor explanations in the *MSMR* for such large changes. Given the importance of the data, anyone interested in the data would certainly want to understand the nature of the changes. It is not simply implausible, but defies belief that such a shift would take place in such a casual manner.

What is going on here? Did someone realize certain types of adverse events were already spiking in 2021, and did they tamper with previous years' data to make the spike look smaller?

And why did the revisions affect only ambulatory cases? Crawford suggests that hospital data may be harder to tamper with, due to standardization of reporting systems.

These findings were huge—suggestive of data tampering on a massive scale.

And, as Crawford would later point out, the server migration that DoD claimed took place in August of 2021 would have been an ideal opportunity to wipe clean the fingerprints of any data tampering operation.

Shamefully, this story has been completely ignored by the legacy media.

A Grossly Inadequate Response

The very next day, Senator Johnson dispatched yet another message, this time to Health and Human Services Secretary Xavier Becerra along with

FDA Commissioner Robert Califf, NIAID Director Anthony Fauci, and CDC Director Rochelle Walensky. The senator did not mince words:

> To date, I have written 35 letters to the Executive Branch asking questions relating to the COVID-19 pandemic and the federal government's response to it. The grossly inadequate response to my legitimate oversight demonstrates a level of arrogance to the American public that is unacceptable.
>
> The extent to which federal health agencies have ignored the vaccine safety signals coming from the Vaccine Adverse Event Reporting System (VAERS) is mind-boggling. As of March 18, 2022, VAERS has received 1,183,495 worldwide reports of adverse events and 25,641 death reports. Of those deaths, 7,382 occurred on day 0, 1, or 2 following vaccination.

Senator Johnson went on to point out that the previous month, Andreas Schofbeck, a board member of BKK ProVita, a German health insurance company that insures over eleven million people, had stated that BKK customers had reported 216,000 adverse reactions to the covid vaccines, according to the data that was available for 2021. Extrapolating from this figure, Schofbeck estimated that as many as three million Germans had received medical treatment for adverse reactions to the shot, a figure that dwarfed the estimated 246,000 vaccine adverse reactions reported to the Paul Erlich Institute (the German equivalent of the CDC). This would mean that something like only eight percent of vaccine-related adverse events were being reported, for an under-reporting factor of twelve or more.

Schofbeck was dismissed from his post after making his concerns public.

The epistle also mentioned the staggering rise in the death rate of working-age adults OneAmerica CEO Scott Davison had called attention to the previous January, and the shocking safety signals whistleblowers had obtained from DMED.

Senator Johnson had a number of questions for the recipients of his message, among which were:

- Is your agency aware of Mr. Schofbeck's February 2022 letter and BKK ProVita data regarding potential significant underreporting of COVID-19 vaccine adverse events in Germany?

- What has your agency undertaken to determine whether U.S. insurance companies have seen increases in claims filed relating to COVID-19 vaccine adverse events over the last year? What has your agency found? If your agency has not made any determination, please explain why not.

- What has your agency undertaken to determine whether U.S. insurance companies have seen increases in claims filed relating to non-COVID-19 deaths among 18 to 64 year olds over the last year? What has your agency found? If your agency has not made any determination, please explain why not.

- Are you concerned by the adverse events reported in VAERS associated with COVID-19 vaccination? If so, please explain what steps, if any, you are taking to address those reports. If not, why are 1,183,495 reports of adverse events associated with vaccination not a concern to you?

The senator requested the agencies reply to his concerns no later than 6 April.

The next day, New York City Mayor Eric Adams announced that unvaccinated professional athletes and performers would be exempted from the ban preventing them from working in that city. In response to the glad tidings, CBS New York gushed "It means Nets fans can soon see Kyrie Irving play home games and that a full roster of players can take the field when the Mets and Yankees open their seasons."[313]

Her Anti-Vaccination and Anti-Government Views
are Unmistakable

On 7 April, an Israeli study showed that the effectiveness of a *fourth* dose of the mRNA vaccine in preventing infection by the Omicron variant faded rapidly, to a paltry thirty percent after thirty-three days in the case of the Pfizer vax, and an even punier eleven percent after just twenty-three days for the Moderna product. The researchers attempted to put the best possible spin on these findings, concluding "Our data provide evidence that a fourth dose of mRNA is immunogenic, safe, and somewhat efficacious."[314]

Fifteen days later, Pfizer filed a motion in the Eastern District Court of Texas requesting that Brook Jackson's whistleblower suit be dismissed. The very first page of the motion contains these words:

> The U.S. Department of Defense ("DoD") has purchased every one of these shots and provided them to Americans at no cost.

That was an odd statement, given that the taxpayers had handed over $1.95 billion to Pfizer for the first hundred million doses, and billions of dollars after that. Perhaps Pfizer's lawyers meant to say "… no cost *at the point of delivery.*" But never mind that for now.

The motion to dismiss was based on a 2016 Supreme Court decision which stated that "If the government pays a particular claim in full despite its actual knowledge that certain requirements were violated, that is very strong evidence that those requirements were not material." The motion went on to argue that since the Pfizer shots were purchased by the Department of Defense under its "Other Transaction Authority," the sale was not subject to the Federal Acquisition Regulation which governs most transactions with appropriated funds.

Not content to let matters rest there, Pfizer's lawyers proceed to let us know the kind of woman we are dealing with here:

Her anti-vaccination and anti-Government views are unmistakable. For example, she has tweeted that "there's no way in Hell [she] would let a Covid jab" near her children, even though the CDC recommends that vaccine for everyone 5 years of age and older.

She has said the entire Government is "complicit in a scheme to hide the truth" and "complicit in fraud, period." And she has called Dr. Anthony Fauci, the Director of the National Institute of Allergies and Infectious Disease ("NIAID") both "scary" and "the face of corruption and evil."

The Information in This Document is Proprietary and Confidential

On the first of May, an interesting finding emerged from the Pfizer data dump. The document began with this advisory:

> The information contained in this document is proprietary and confidential. Any disclosure, reproduction, distribution, or other dissemination of this information outside of Pfizer, its Affiliates, its Licensees, or Regulatory Agencies is strictly prohibited. Except as may be otherwise agreed to in writing, by accepting or reviewing these materials, you agree to hold such information in confidence and not to disclose it to others (except where required by applicable law), nor to use it for unauthorized purposes.

What was the reason for these rather ominous words of warning? Perhaps the answer can be found on page six, wherein it was revealed that the company had been flooded with so many adverse event reports they had to hire the equivalent of an additional six hundred full-time employees to process them, with an expected total of more than eighteen hundred to be "onboarded" by June of 2021.

Dumpster Diving and Playing Footsie

Later that month another controversy arose regarding a widely shared claim on social media that the Pfizer vaccine was only "twelve percent effective." This figure appeared to have arisen in a Substack post by Sonja Elijah,[315] a reporter who also writes for *Trial Site News*. The claim arose from the FDA briefing document that had actually been in the public domain since December of 2020—long before the Pfizer data dump commenced. The website FullFact rated the story as "inaccurate."[316]

Elijah arrived at the figure of twelve percent efficacy by dividing the number of cases of "suspected covid" (1,594) in the treatment arm by the number in the placebo arm (1,816) and subtracting the result from one. But she made a basic miscalculation, neglecting the cases of confirmed covid in the placebo arm (162 cases) and the treatment arm (eight cases). The correct calculation would be 1 - (1,594+8)/(1,816+162), to get the (still underwhelming) figure of nineteen percent efficacy against covid-like symptoms that Dr. Doshi had arrived at more than a year previously in his essay in *BMJ Blogs*. So again, the fact checkers had a point.

Dr. Gorski of Science-Based Medicine joined the fray,[317] pointing out the flaws in Elijah's figure of twelve percent effectiveness (Jeffrey Morris, Professor of Biostatistics at the Perlman School of Medicine at the University of Pennsylvania had already made the same arguments in a blog post four days previously).[318] Gorski called the twelve percent figure a "slasher stat," "so-named because it is not new and like the killers in slasher movie series, even when it appears to be dead it always appears in another installment of the misinformation franchise to kill again."[319]

Dr. Gorski goes on to point out that the Pfizer trial protocol called for all participants experiencing symptoms of COVID-19 to report for either an in-person or telehealth visit and be tested. This is true so far as it goes, but it ignores that fact that cases of covid occurring up to twenty-eight days after the first shot were not counted toward the primary endpoint. How many such cases were there? Once again, if Gorski has any idea, he isn't saying.

Dr. Gorski then lays the blame squarely at the feet of Dr. Doshi:

> The BMJ published an article that used exactly the same massively flawed rationale to downplay the efficacy of the Pfizer vaccine that antivaxxers are using now. Worse, it continues to employ the author of that commentary, Peter Doshi, as an associate editor.
>
> Worse, the BMJ hired Doshi despite his long history of playing footsie with the antivaccine movement since at least 2009, amplifying antivaccine conspiracy theories, downplaying the severity of influenza and thus feeding antivaccine narratives.
>
> He's only gotten worse since the COVID-19 pandemic. For example, he's used his title as BMJ editor when taking part in a "roundtable" organized by Sen. Ron Johnson to go dumpster diving in VAERS to find "vaccine injuries" due to COVID-19 vaccines, whether the injuries were caused by them or not.
>
> In a truly risible moment, he even cited the Merriam-Webster definition of "antivaxxer" as opposed to those supposedly opposed to vaccine mandates to argue that he and his fellow COVID-19 contrarians were "not antivaccine."
>
> He even parroted the antivaccine talking point that mRNA vaccines are not really vaccines and therefore shouldn't be mandated like vaccines.[320]

On 23 May, the Department of Health and Human Services recommended a third (booster) shot of the Pfizer vax for persons between five and eleven years of age, and a fourth (second booster) shot for individuals over the age of fifty as well as immunocompromised patients between the ages of twelve and forty-nine.[321]

Five days later, my Facebook account was restricted for posting "false information about COVID-19 that goes against our community standards." Every bit of information in the offending post had been taken from VAERS.

CHAPTER ELEVEN

The Plot Thickens

June–August 2022

The Smoking Gun?

On Wednesday 8 June, what may turn out to be the smoking gun in this case was revealed. Writing in his Substack, documentary producer Phil Harper drew attention to a tweet from a Twitter user who styles himself "Jikkyleaks" regarding a file with the inauspicious name adva.zip, released on 1 May as part of the Pfizer data dump.[322]

We have already mentioned that any cases of COVID-19 occurring in the first twenty-eight days of the trial were not counted toward the primary endpoint. We don't know how many cases went uncounted, but now we have a clue.

Apparently, Pfizer took blood samples from all patients in the trial, and tested them for antibodies against the nucleocapsid protein contained in the outer membrane of the virus (N-Antibodies). This is important, because the shot does not stimulate production of these antibodies—meaning that anyone manifesting such antibodies must have been infected with the coronavirus.

Jikkyleaks claimed to have found the following results:

N-Antibodies Visit 1	N-Antibodies Visit 3	BNT162b	Placebo
Positive	Positive	343	377
Negative	Negative	15,914	15,708
Negative	Positive	75	160
Positive	Negative	18	18

So, the vast majority of patients tested (about sixteen thousand in each arm of the trial) were negative for N-antibodies at the start of the trial. That means they never had been infected.

Of these, 160 patients in the placebo arm seroconverted—meaning they went on to produce N-antibodies, demonstrating they had been infected—as opposed to seventy-five in the treatment arm. If this be true, the effectiveness of the Pfizer shot in preventing covid infections is about fifty-four percent—barely within the range needed to be considered "effective," according to the FDA.

It gets worse. A study released in preprint form the previous April which utilized data from the trial of the Moderna shot—which, as you should recall, forces the body to produce the exact same protein as the Pfizer product—looked at patients with PCR-confirmed COVID-19 infection. Only forty percent of the subjects in the treatment arm had measurable levels of N-antibodies, as opposed to ninety-three percent in the placebo arm.[323] So we may expect that the figure of seventy-five patients in the treatment arm who went on to become infected with COVID-19 underestimated the actual number by a factor of more than two.

In plain English, the much-vaunted figure of "ninety percent efficacy" for the Pfizer shot was now looking more like zero percent. Maybe even negative efficacy.

How can this be? We have already seen there is ample evidence that the vax *increases* the likelihood of covid infection in the first two weeks or more after administration of the first shot, perhaps by depressing the production of lymphocytes. Those cases were not counted, presumably on the grounds that patients had not had time to develop immunity to the spike protein. But what on earth difference does this make to the patient, who presumably wants to know only one thing: will this shot decrease the likelihood of my contracting COVID-19, or will it not? Whether the infection occurs within the first two weeks after the first shot or sometime after should make no difference at all.

At the time of my writing this (22 July 2022), the Twitter account @ Jikkyleaks was suspended. Fortunately, the relevant document can readily be obtained on the PHMPT website. This file weighs in at a whopping 170 megabytes (for calibration, that's approximately eighty-five time the size of Tolstoy's *War and Peace*) but Harper provided detailed instructions for downloading the file and extracting the relevant information, and claimed to have obtained the exact same figures as Jikkyleaks.

This was huge. Hundreds of millions of people worldwide had been induced or coerced into having Pfizer's experimental gene therapy shot into their bodies and now, it seemed, this product provided no reduction in the Pfizer trial's primary endpoint—covid infection of any severity.

Shamefully, this story has been completely ignored by the legacy media.

Unissant Does Not Have Access to These Documents

Six days later, Senator Ron Johnson dispatched a letter to Kenneth Bonner, President and Chief Growth Officer of Unissant, regarding the shocking safety signals pertaining to the covid vax contained in DMED. The senator stated that data downloaded from DMED and provided to his office by whistleblowers on 29 August 2021 showed a total of 216 cases of myocarditis for the years 2016-2020 inclusive, for an average of 43.2 cases per year, while the total for 2021 was 1,239—a whopping 2,868 percent increase (and the year wasn't even over yet). On 10 January 2022, newly downloaded data showed the total reported cases for 2016-2020 rose from 216 to 559, or 111.8 per year, while total cases for 2021 dropped from 1,239 to 263. Thus the reported increase in cases for 2021 dropped from a staggering 2,868 percent to a (still concerning) 235 percent. These data were provided to the senator's office on 23 January—the day before the meeting of the expert panel.

As we have already noted, Senator Johnson had contacted Unissant and demanded an explanation, and Unissant had refused. After an exchange of emails between the senator's office, Unissant, and DoD, on 4 May Unissant provided responsive documents to the senator's request.

The documents did not settle all the questions raised by Senator Johnson, and in fact raised some new ones. Specifically, the senator demanded to know:

- Why the DMED data for registered diagnoses of certain medical conditions from 2016-2020 were incorrect

- Why registered diagnoses of myocarditis in 2021 decreased from 1,239 as of 29 August 2021 to 263 as of 10 January 2022

- Why registered diagnoses of myocarditis from the period 2016-2020 increased from 216 to 559

Finally, Senator Johnson pointed out that Unissant's response of 4 May claimed that because its employees use DoD email addresses when communicating with that department, "Unissant does not have access to those documents and communications." The senator wanted to know how Unissant ensures that its employees are following federal record preservation records if the company cannot access communications by its own employees.

The senator requested the agencies reply to his concerns no later than 28 June.

Lowering the Bar

On 18 June, the Department of Health and Human Services approved the two-dose series of the Moderna vax for children between the ages of six months through five years, along with a third (booster) dose for immuno-compromised children, and the three-dose series of the Pfizer shot for children aged six months through four years.[324]

An article that ran in the *New York Times*[325] the following day showed how the bar had been progressively lowered for that kind of thing. In contrast to the over ninety percent efficacy figures originally touted for these nostrums (and always remember, that figure referred to relative reduction in risk, not absolute reduction), Moderna's data showed an efficacy of just fifty-one percent for tots between the ages of six through twenty-three months, and an even more paltry thirty-seven percent for those aged two through five years. Meanwhile, Pfizer, which already had failed even to meet the FDA criteria for immune response for the two-dose series, was now claiming an efficacy rate of eighty percent for the three-dose regimen. But that figure was based on a total of just three cases in the treatment arm of the trial versus seven in the placebo arm.

The process of lowering of the bar continued. Eight days later, another *NYT* article reported that both Pfizer and Moderna were working on a new iteration of their product which targeted new subvariants of the Omicron variant of SARS-CoV-2. (Up to this point, booster shots had not been tailored to new variants, but were nothing more than repeat shots of the same old formulation targeting the original Wuhan strain, which had long since come and gone.) Unfortunately, the article stated, "The virus is evolving so quickly that new vaccine formulations are out of date before such trials are even finished," concluding "This suggests that officials would have to base their judgements largely on animal trials and laboratory tests."[326]

Four days after that, yet another *NYT* article stated that the Department of Health and Human Services had agreed to pay out $3.2 billion to

Pfizer and BioNTech to purchase an additional 105 million doses of the vax, with an option to buy up to three hundred million doses. The article also quoted Dr. Offit, who noted that Pfizer and BioNTech had yet to share any data that demonstrated the reformulated version increases the chances of being protected against severe disease.[327]

Data Mining Is Outside of the Agency's Purview

Meanwhile, on the twenty-third of that month, Senator Johnson dispatched a message to CDC Director Rochelle Walensky regarding the center's failure to carry out promised signal detection analysis of VAERS data.

As you should recall, the center's Standard Operating Procedures (SOP) for COVID-19, released 29 January 2021, mandated the agency would carry out Proportional Report Ratio analysis of VAERS data weekly. The SOP also stipulated that the FDA would conduct a more sophisticated analysis of vaccine-associated adverse events, called empirical Bayesian data mining, on a biweekly basis. All this had been re-affirmed in the updated SOP released 2 February 2022.

A Freedom of Information Act request filed 9 May by Children's Health Defense elicited this reply from the CDC:

> No PRR's were conducted by the CDC.
>
> Data mining is outside of the agency's purview.
>
> While VAERS has conducted "signal assessment" as described in section 2.5 (i.e. assessed that a causal association exists between the vaccine and both TTS [Thrombosis with Thrombocytopenia Syndrome] and myocarditis), that assessment involved no formal records.

The missive did not explain what it means to perform an "assessment" which involves "no formal records."

Senator Johnson requested the center hand over all documents requested in the FOIA request, adding "If CDC did not collect any of the above information, please explain why and detail who made the decision to not follow the SOP and when that decision was made."

The senator requested the agencies reply to his concerns no later than 7 July.

The American People Deserve the Truth

On Friday 8 July I visited my primary care provider—a local semi-celebrity whose services I retained after he had reached out to me to express admiration for a couple of op-ed pieces I had published in the *Baltimore Sun*—and he agreed to write a letter exempting me from having to take any more booster shots. That was one fewer worry on my mind.

That same day, the *New York Times* reported that the rates of COVID-19 infections and hospitalizations were climbing once more, even in countries with high vaccination rates, as the new subvariants BA.4 and BA.5 became dominant.[328] The piece began with this interesting bit of spin: "The most transmissible variant yet of the coronavirus is threatening a fresh wave of infections in the United States, even among those who have recovered from the virus fairly recently." The ability of the virus to infect the vaccinated was not mentioned until four paragraphs later.

Thirteen days later, the *Epoch Times* reported that two state attorneys general—Eric Schmitt of Missouri and Jeff Landry of Louisiana—had filed a suit alleging Anthony Fauci and other government officials had conspired to suppress information regarding the covid pandemic.[329] Dr. Fauci was ordered to turn over all communications with a variety of social media platforms related to the Great Barrington Declaration. He was also instructed to identify every worker in his administration who had communicated with a social media platform regarding "content modulation" and/or misinformation.

The suit named a number of other current and former government officials, including White House Press Secretary Karine Jean-Pierre as well as Nina Jankowicz, the erstwhile head of the ill-fated "Disinformation Governance Board."

On that same day, a team of from Brigham and Women's Hospital and Massachusetts General Hospital reported in the *New England Journal of Medicine* that the duration of viral shedding after PCR-confirmed covid infection was exactly the same for vaccinated and unvaccinated subjects, and in fact was *longer* for those who had their booster shot.[330]

Also on that same day—exactly one year after President Biden told the nation "You're not going to get covid if you've had these vaccinations," the White House announced that the president, after being double-vaxxed and double-boosted, had been diagnosed with COVID-19.[331]

Ashish Jha, White House Covid Response Coordinator, assured reporters:

> The President is doing better. He slept well last night. He ate his breakfast and lunch—fully. He actually showed me his plate![332]

Two days later, the *Epoch Times* reported that John Su, head of the VAERS team at the CDC, had told them in an email that the CDC had been performing Proportional Report Ratio analysis since February of 2021 and was continuing to do so. This was in direct contradiction to what the Children's Health Defense had reported the CDC had said in response to its Freedom of Information Act request of 9 May.[333]

Two days after that, Senator Johnson fired off yet another missive to CDC Director Rochelle Walensky. The senator noted that the agency had failed to respond to the previous oversight letter of 23 June which was sent in response to the allegations made by Children's Health Defense, that the CDC had told them "No PRR's were performed" and "data mining is outside of the agency's purview."

In a scathing dispatch, the senator wrote:

> The American people deserve the truth and you have not been providing it. That is why I, together with millions of Americans, have completely lost faith in the CDC and other federal health agencies.
>
> Accordingly, please provide an immediate and complete response to my June 23, 2022 letter and the following information by no later than July 29, 2022:
>
> 1) Is Dr. Su's statement that "CDC has been performing PRRs since Feb 2021, and continues to do so to date" true?
>   a) If so, why did CDC claim that "No PRRs were conducted" in response to a May 9 FOIA request?
>   b) If Dr. Su's statement is true, please provide all of the PRRs performed since February 2021.
> 2) Please make Dr. Su available for an interview with my office to discuss the types of surveillance CDC has performed regarding COVID-19 vaccine adverse events and the data CDC has generated based on its surveillance.

A Red Herring

Two days later, an article in the *New York Times* reported that a survey by the Kaiser Family Foundation found significant reluctance on the part of parents to have their young children vaccinated. Forty-three percent of parents of children under the age of five years told pollsters they would "definitely not" have their little ones vaxxed, while twenty-seven percent said they would "wait and see" and another thirteen percent would have their children get the shot "only if required."[334]

The article also contained the requisite pithy quotes from experts:

Although the vast majority of children who come down with Covid get over it easily, "some kids get very ill from it and some die," said Patricia A. Stinchfield, the president of the National Foundation for Infectious Diseases.

Dr. Jason V. Terk, a pediatrician in Keller, Texas, acknowledged "the reality" that the extremely contagious Omicron subvariant BA.5 "is evading both natural immunity and vaccination immunity much more than the other variants." Still, he said, "The vaccine is the best way to protect younger children from the occasions in which Covid-19 causes more severe illness."

This sort of argument is an old red herring tactic, deftly evading the question of whether a given intervention reduces all-cause mortality or all serious adverse events.

Two days after that, another *NYT* article reported that enthusiasm for booster shots was waning almost as rapidly as the efficacy of those shots. While half of adults eligible for their first booster received one, only thirty percent of those eligible for their second booster did likewise. The piece also mentioned that the FDA had decided that those under fifty years of age should hold off on getting boosted until the reformulated version of the shot—intended to provide superior protection against the new BA.5 subvariant—became available in early September.[335]

On 2 August, the New Civil Liberties Alliance announced it was joining Missouri and Louisiana in their lawsuit against President Biden, Anthony Fauci, the CDC, and a number of other federal agencies and officials, alleging that they had conspired to suppress freedom of speech regarding covid vaccines and treatments on a variety of social media platforms. Two of the three authors of the Great Barrington Declaration—Martin Kulldorff and Jay Bhattacharya—had also joined the suit, as did Aaron Kheriaty, who had been fired from his position at UC Irvine Medical School for refusing the vax.

Five days later, Pfizer announced it would spend $5.4 billion to buy the biotech firm Global Blood Therapeutics. This deal came in the wake of the drugmaker's $11.6 billion acquisition of Biohaven and it $6.7 billion purchase of Arena Pharmaceuticals.[336]

Two days after that, the CDC issued its revised guidelines for dealing with the pandemic.[337] Gone were the totally unworkable anti-social distancing rules which not one human being on the planet had observed consistently anyway. The agency also acknowledged the painfully obvious: that previous infection with COVID-19 reduces the risk of future infections. In addition, the new guidelines no longer called for universal masking, or testing of asymptomatic people.

Instead, the guidelines included this rather tepid endorsement of the benefits of repeated booster shots:

> Being up to date with vaccination provides a transient period of increased protection against infection and transmission after the most recent dose, although protection can wane over time.

Again they repeated a by-now familiar red herring argument:

> The rates of COVID-19-associated hospitalization and death are substantially higher among unvaccinated adults than among those who are up-to-date with recommended COVID-19 vaccination, particularly adults aged > 65 years.

As we have seen, this is a formulation that ignores the only outcomes that matter—all cause hospitalizations or deaths. The guidelines also neglected to mention that deaths occurring in the "partially vaccinated" (i.e. within the first four weeks after the first does of the Pfizer shot, or the first six weeks after the first dose of the Moderna vax) are not counted toward this endpoint.[338]

Emerging evidence suggests that vaccination before infection also provides some protection against post-COVID-19 conditions.

What was the "emerging evidence" for this statement? The CDC didn't say.

Overall booster dose coverage in the United States remains low, which is concerning given the meaningful reductions in risk for severe illness and death that booster doses provide and the importance of booster doses to counter waning of vaccine-induced immunity.

The CDC didn't mention who found this concerning. Obviously not the millions of Americans who are forgoing these booster shots.

All in all, the public seemed to greet these guidelines with a yawn, as an attempt by the CDC to get out in front of the changes that were going to occur with or without the CDC's guidance, as increasing numbers of Americans grew tired of being governed by fear and started taking back their lives.

At this point it should be obvious to all that the covid "vaccines" are not "vaccines" at all, at least as the word has been understood to mean for more than a century. They are, at best, therapeutics which must be administered in advance of the infection, with a limited window of efficacy, and a terrible side effects profile. How can we even think about mandating these products?

Four days later Pfizer CEO Albert Bourla, who had already been double-vaxxed and double-boosted, announced that he had been infected with the covid.[339]

On 24 August, a press release was issued by Cedars Sinai of Los Angeles titled "New Data Show COVID-19 Vaccine Does Not Raise Stroke Risk." The piece quoted Alexis Simpkins, Director of Vascular Neurology Research at Cedars Sinai:

You're 200 times less likely—if you compare the numbers—to have had a stroke if you were vaccinated, than a person who was hospitalized with severe COVID-19 and was not vaccinated.[340]

This was a breathtakingly mendacious argument, akin to comparing all the drunk drivers in the country with sober drivers who had already been hospitalized in an ICU for car crash injuries, and then concluding that drunk driving is safer than sober driving.

Three days later, the *New York Times* reported that Moderna was suing Pfizer and BioNTech for patent infringement regarding the mRNA vaccines.[341] Experts predicted the litigation could drag on for years.

On the last day of the month, the California State Assembly approved AB 2098, a bill which would designate "dissemination of misinformation or disinformation related to COVID-19 as "unprofessional conduct." The bill defined "misinformation" as "false information that is contradicted by contemporary scientific consensus," and "disinformation" as "misinformation that the licensee deliberately disseminated with malicious intent or an intent to mislead."

Rigorous Safety and Effectiveness Standards

That same day, the FDA announced it had granted Emergency Use Authorization to both Pfizer's and Moderna's new "bivalent" booster shots, reformulated to give protection against the BA.4 and BA.5 variants of Omicron (both of which have the exact same spike protein amino acid sequence) as well as the original Wuhan strain—which had already come and gone.[342] The new reformulated version was never even tested for safety and efficacy in human subjects—although, in fairness, it should be mentioned that the previous June, Pfizer had presented preliminary data on the effects of the shot in eight mice.[343] Instead, the FDA relied on data from trials of another version of the shot, engineered to give protection against the BA.1 variant which, like the Wuhan strain, had also already come and gone.[344]

Peter Marks, Director of the FDA Center for Biological Evaluation Research, stated:

> The public can be assured that a great deal of care has been taken by the FDA to ensure these bivalent COVID-19 vaccines meet our rigorous safety, effectiveness and manufacturing quality standards for emergency use authorization.[345]

Not everyone shared his enthusiasm. Dr. Offit, one of only two members of the FDA advisory panel to have voted against the EUA, told the *New York Times* that the incubation period for COVID-19 was too short for the vaccines to have any effect on the course of the pandemic:

> Even if 100% of the population were vaccinated and the virus hadn't evolved at all, vaccines would do very little to stop transmission.[346]

Filtering out the Noise

The same day the FDA granted the EUA for the new bivalent booster shots, Dr. Doshi and several of his colleagues published an analysis of serious adverse events of special interest in the Pfizer and Moderna trials, using a list of such events that had been compiled previously by the Brighton Collaboration, a global authority on the topic of vaccine safety, and endorsed by the World Health Organization Global Advisory Committee on Vaccine Safety.[347]

What makes a serious adverse event of "special interest?" Well, the list includes serious adverse events believed to be associated with the mRNA platform as well as those associated with vaccines in general, theoretical associations based on animal models, and—most importantly—those known to be caused by the coronavirus.

Dr. Doshi explained the reasoning behind all this to me:

> So what it does is, in effect, is that it filters out those things
> for which associations are less likely to exist. So therefore it
> filters out the noise. Right? Because there's always noise in
> data. There's always background. That's why there's serious
> adverse events that occur in the placebo group.
>
> We took one filter, which is adverse events of special
> interest, to try and get something that was more sensitive to
> detecting a signal if a signal exists.

Dr. Doshi and his co-authors found the Pfizer and Moderna products
were associated with one additional serious adverse event of special interest
for every eight hundred individuals vaccinated. Ninety-seven percent of
these events were known to be associated with the pathogenesis of the
coronavirus itself. The most common of the elevated serious adverse events
were "coagulation events," a category that includes blood clots and ischemic
stroke. All serious adverse events increased as well, by thirty-six percent.
And yes, the difference was statistically significant.

An increase of six percent was reported for the Moderna vaccine, but
for reasons the authors explain, this is probably an underestimate due to
the way Moderna reported its trial results. Only detailed raw data will
allow for such an assessment and to date, neither the company nor the
FDA has released the data.

Granted, the one in eight hundred increase in AESI's may seem small,
but multiply that by hundreds of millions of people who have been given
these shots and you have a problem. (For calibration, according to the
Department of Health and Human Services, the rate of serious allergic
reactions to other vaccines is on the order or one to two per *million*.)[348]
Also, keep in mind these trials were slated to go on for two years but
were shut down after barely seven percent of the patients made it to the

six-month mark. What happens after that? Nobody who is in a position to find out seems interested in doing so.

The authors also pointed out that waning vaccine effectiveness, decreased viral virulence, and increasing immune escape from vaccines would further shift the balance in the harms-benefit equation in the direction of harm, and factors that lower the risk for complications due to COVID-19—i.e. natural immunity, younger age, and lack of comorbidities—would shift the balance further still.

What do you call a "medicine" that creates more problems than it solves?

A poison.

CHAPTER TWELVE

What About Long Covid?

As the evidence continues to mount for the harms and lack of efficacy of the shots, and as ever-increasing numbers of us grow tired of being governed by fear, the Mandators have one last ace in the hole to play: the specter of Long Covid.

"Long Covid has resulted in a 'mass disabling event,'" the *Los Angeles Times* intoned ominously,[349] while the *Wall Street Journal* informed readers "Between two million and four million Americans aren't working due to the long-term effects of Covid-19."[350]

All this raises a question: just what is "Long Covid?"

On 5 May 2020, Paul Garner, Professor of Infectious Diseases at the Liverpool School of Tropical Medicine described his experience with COVID-19 in a post in *BMJ Blogs*:

> For almost seven weeks I have been through a roller coaster of ill health, extreme emotions, and utter exhaustion.[351]

Dr. Garner, a former military physician and fitness enthusiast before his illness, found himself besieged by a variety of complaints: malaise, tachycardia, tightness in the chest, "muggy head," upset stomach, tinnitus, aches, dyspnea, arthritis, and more. He also told of joining a Facebook group where he met patients like himself, struggling to understand what was happening:

People suffering from the disease, but not believing their symptoms were real; their families thinking the symptoms were anxiety; employers telling people they had to return to work, as the two weeks for the illness was up.[352]

Elise Perego, a researcher at the University College Institute of Archeology and sufferer of this condition, is believed to have coined the term "long covid," which she first used as a Twitter hashtag on 20 May of that year.[353] The first use of this term in the popular press was in a 25 June article in Sky News, which told the tale of Jake Suett, an ICU doctor in Norfolk who first developed symptoms earlier that year. What started out as tiredness and a sore throat soon turned into fever, dry cough, and shortness of breath. Twelve weeks later he was suffering from chest pain, breathlessness, blurred vision, memory loss, poor concentration, gastrointestinal symptoms, and shooting pains in his hands and feet, and was unable to return to work.[354] The next month, the term was used for the first time in a medical journal, in an article in the *BMJ*.[355]

On 6 October 2021, the World Health Organization issued a definition of something called "post-COVID-19 Condition":

> Post COVID-19 condition occurs in individuals with a history of probable or confirmed SARS CoV-2 infection, usually 3 months from the onset of COVID-19 with symptoms and that last for at least 2 months and cannot be explained by an alternative diagnosis. Common symptoms include fatigue, shortness of breath, cognitive dysfunction but also others and generally have an impact on everyday functioning. Symptoms may be new onset following initial recovery from an acute COVID-19 episode or persist from the initial illness. Symptoms may also fluctuate or relapse over time.[356]

This syndrome has also been dubbed long-haul covid, post-acute COVID-19, post-acute sequelae of SARS CoV-2 infection, long term effects of covid, and chronic covid, but "long covid" seems to be the preferred term, and that is the one we shall use here.

Whatever you call it, the syndrome encompasses a vast variety of complaints, involving every organ system in the body along with systemic reactions such as fatigue, post-exertional malaise, fever, chills, skin sensations, weakness, night sweats—the list goes on and on. A study by British and American researchers and patient advocates listed sixty-six different symptoms and found the mean time to recovery exceeded thirty-five weeks.[357] Another study by British researchers described three recurring symptom clusters in patients with this condition: a cardiopulmonary syndrome manifesting with exertional intolerance, dyspnea, fatigue, autonomic dysfunction, tachycardia, lung abnormalities, and chest pain; a multi-organ syndrome comprising general autoimmune activation and a proinflammatory state along with gastrointestinal symptoms, dermatological symptoms, and fever; and a neuropsychiatric syndrome including brain fog, dizziness, poor memory and cognition, mood disorders, headache, and chronic pain.[358] Yet another British study found the risk factors for long covid were pretty much what you'd expect them to be: smoking, obesity, a wide range of comorbid conditions, and ethnic minority status. Perhaps surprisingly, age was not a risk factor, once all these other factors were controlled.[359]

The CDC guidelines[360] (revised 1 September 2022) stipulate that these is no test for long covid, and that the same symptoms can come from any of a variety of other health problems. Estimates of the prevalence of this condition in post-infection patients range from three percent to fifty.

It's not a foregone conclusion that all cases of "long covid" have a common cause. Many studies employ a rather liberal definition of this condition (e.g., persistence of one or more symptoms after twelve weeks). And there is no way of knowing how many of these complaints might be due to any of the myriad underlying conditions which are known risk factors for this diagnosis. Still, there doesn't seem to be any doubt that we're dealing with a real syndrome here, in at least some cases.

Fortunately, we are told, help is on the way. A March 2022 article in *Lancet Respiratory Medicine* stated "There are encouraging emerging data that individuals who are vaccinated against COVID-19 are less likely to report long covid symptoms."[361] The CDC guidelines advise "Research suggests that people who are vaccinated but experience a breakthrough infection are less likely to report post-covid conditions."[362]

The trope has been dutifully picked up by the legacy media:

> "Research is showing that people who are vaccinated, even with just one dose, tend to have lower rates of long COVID-19 after catching the virus than those who are unvaccinated." (National Public Radio)[363]

> "Vaccinations and boosters are believed to be helpful at staving off long covid." (Los Angeles Times)[364]

> "Not only will a booster with the new vaccines decrease the likelihood of infection and severe illness and help reduce transmission of the virus; it could also decrease the likelihood of developing long Covid." (New York Times)[365]

So does the vax really reduce the chances of long covid? Researchers at the Department of Veterans Affairs (which administers the largest nationally integrated healthcare delivery system in the United States) looked at VA records and concluded that cases of long covid arising through breakthrough infections was reduced compared to that of a group of never-vaccinated matched controls by all of fifteen percent.[366] That works out to a less than one in five hundred reduction in absolute risk.

And there is no way of knowing how much of that paltry reduction in risk is due to clinician bias. Remember, "long covid" is a diagnosis of exclusion. Could it be doctors are less likely to attribute a patient's complaints to "long covid" if that patient has already been vaxxed?

Anyway, it's all a moot point. No one is denying the people manifesting the most extreme presentations of this syndrome are suffering. No one is denying these are serious adverse events. These patients deserve our compassion and the very best care modern medicine has to offer.

But all this begs the question of whether the shot reduces the frequency of the only outcome that matters—all serious adverse events. And we have already seen that Pfizer's and Moderna's data—the data they have let us see—shows it does not.

And that's in the short term. We don't know what the long-term harms of these products are. We had a golden opportunity to find out, but as we have also already seen, the trials were cut short by the drugmakers long before they were slated to end.

In the light of all this, efforts to terrify us into getting endless boosters by waving the bloody shirt of "long covid" are the height of mendacity.

CHAPTER THIRTEEN

Disinformation

September 2022

Be on the Lookout

On the first day of September, Aaron Kheriaty, who had been fired from his position at the UC Irvine Medical School for refusing the shot, updated the readers of his Substack on the progress of *Missouri v Biden*, the lawsuit filed by the attorneys general of Missouri and Louisiana against President Biden along with numerous other officials and agencies for allegedly conspiring to suppress freedom of speech on matters related to the covid pandemic on a variety of social media platforms.[367]

Through the process of discovery, the plaintiffs had determined that scores of officials from at least eleven different federal agencies had communicated with social media platforms to suppress private speech the officials disfavored. The agencies involved included the White House, Health and Human Services, Homeland Security, the CDC, the FDA, NIAID, the Census Bureau, the State Department, the Treasury Department, the US Election Assistance Commission, and the Cybersecurity and Infrastructure Security Agency (CISA).

At least thirty-two federal officials had communicated with Meta (owner of both Facebook and Instagram) about its content. Eleven federal officials had communicated with YouTube, and nine had communicated with Twitter.

The findings provided revealing glimpses into the pressure that had been put on the operators of these social media platforms. After President Biden had publicly said of Facebook on 16 July 2021 "They're killing people," a senior executive at Meta had reached out to Surgeon General Vivek Murthy to engage in damage control and find a way to appease the president's wrath. "It's not great to be accused of killing people" he plainted, adding that he was "keen to find a way to deescalate and work together collaboratively." The same executive contacted Dr. Murthy a week later to assure him that they had removed seventeen pages, groups, and Instagram accounts associated with something called the "Disinfo Dozen," and again a month later to assure Murthy that Facebook "will shortly be expanding our covid policies to further reduce the spread of potentially harmful content," "increasing the strength of our demotions for covid and vaccine-related content," and "making it easier to have Pages/Groups/Accounts demoted for sharing covid and vaccine-related disinformation."

CISA Director Jen Easterly texted another official discussing the importance of "trying to get us into a place where Fed can work with platforms to better understand the mis/dis trends so relevant agencies can try to prebunk/debunk as useful," adding "Platforms have to get more comfortable with gov't. It's really interesting how hesitant they remain."

Officials at Health and Human Services hold weekly "Be on the Lookout" meetings to flag disfavored content; send lists of examples of social media posts to be censored; serve as "fact-checkers" whom social media platforms consult about censoring private speech; and receive detailed reports from social media companies about so-called "misinformation" and "disinformation" activities online.

Dr. Kheriaty wrote:

I suspected all this was happening but didn't imagine the sheer scope—the breadth, depth, and coordination—suggested by the evidence that our legal team has uncovered so far during the discovery phase of the legal proceedings. To see this evidence on the page, which we know is just the tip of the iceberg, is simply shocking.

This evidence suggests we are uncovering the most serious, coordinated, and large-scale violation of First Amendment free speech rights by the federal government's executive branch in U.S. history. Period. Full stop. Even wartime propaganda efforts never reached this level of censorship.

This is Why God Gave Us Two Arms

Five days later, Ashish Jha, White House COVID-19 response coordinator, told reporters:

The good news is that you can get your flu shot and covid shot at the same time. It's actually a good idea.

I really believe this is why God gave us two arms: One for the flu shot and the other one for the covid shot.[368]

Three days after that, FDA Director Robert Califf tweeted:

Being vaccinated or boosted reduces your risk of dying or getting critically ill and going to the hospital. The updated booster also increases your chances of being in attendance at upcoming gatherings with family and friends.

No data were cited in support of these assertions.

An Inadequate and Unacceptable Response

Meanwhile, the story of the CDC's and FDA's dissembling regarding data mining of adverse event reporting continued to become more convoluted. On 12 September, Senator Johnson fired off yet another oversight letter to CDC Director Rochelle Walensky. Some excerpts follow:

> I write to you regarding your inadequate and unacceptable response to my letters about the Centers for Disease Control and Prevention's (CDC) Surveillance of COVID-19 vaccine adverse events. You have failed to explain why the CDC made inconsistent statements about the data it generates to track these adverse events. Moreover, even though I clearly asked CDC to provide the data it supposedly generated to track vaccine adverse events, you failed to do so. This data should be made public immediately to better inform the American people about risks of specific adverse events relating to COVID-19 vaccines.
>
> If CDC is truly conducting proper analyses of COVID-19 vaccine adverse events, it should not take you over two months to provide this information. Accordingly, I ask that you provide complete responses to my June 23 and July 25 letters (enclosed) and the questions below no later than September 19, 2022.
>
> 1) Your response indicated that CDC "recently addressed a previous statement made to the Epoch Times[.]" Was this previous statement connected to Dr. Su's assertion that, "CDC has been performing PRRs since Feb 2021, and continues to do so to date"? If so:
>   a) Was Dr. Su's statement false?
>   b) When and how did CDC address this "previous statement?"

2) Why did CDC misinform the public when it asserted "no PRRs were conducted" and that "data mining is outside of th [sic] agency's purview"? Who at CDC approved the released of this misinformation?

Thank you for your attention to this important matter.

That same day, a study released by researchers at Harvard, the Johns Hopkins University, and other institutions examined the justification for vaccine booster mandates for young adults. Using official data provided by the CDC, the researchers concluded that between 22,000 and 30,000 previously *uninfected* young adults between the ages of eighteen and twenty-nine would have to be boosted to prevent one covid hospitalization—at the cost of anywhere from eighteen to ninety-eight hospitalizations for vaccine-related adverse events.[369] Give that the great majority of people by now *have* been infected, and given that the damage done by the spike protein is dose-related, these figures obviously overestimate the potential benefits and underestimate the potential harms of boosters in this population.

The 2021 Lie of the Year

Two days later, at a hearing convened by the United States Senate Homeland Security and Government Affairs Committee, Senator Johnson questioned current and former executives from Meta, Twitter, YouTube, and Tik Tok on the impact of social media on homeland security.

In methodical, workmanlike fashion, the senator laid out the case against the tech giants which had ruthlessly suppressed official CDC and FDA data on the harms and lack of efficacy of the covid vaccines as "misinformation," and had censored a video of a senate hearing featuring an eminently qualified doctor who had saved the lives of thousands of patients with safe and effective early-stage treatments proven to keep patients alive and out of hospital.

Then Senator Johnson laid it on the line, a rising edge of anger in his voice:

So in July of 2021—talk about misinformation—this should have been the 2021 Lie of the Year: President Biden said "You're not going to get covid if you have these vaccines. If you're vaccinated, you're not going to be hospitalized, you're not going to be in an IC unit, and you're not going to die." That's the President of the United States. Well, it just so happens—we couldn't rely on the CDC and the FDA because they weren't honest and transparent. They weren't giving us data. So we had to go to Public Health England.

This is a chart published from their Technical Briefing Number Twenty-three. It covered the period from February First through September Twelfth, 2021. Five hundred and ninety-three [thousand] cases of mainly Delta, 2,542 deaths, 1,613 deaths occurred with the FULLY VACCINATED. So obviously this was published—and they were publishing other similar information during that time period when President Biden lied to the American public this was a pandemic of the unvaxxed, and if you got vaccinated you're not gonna get— you're not gonna go to the hospital, you're not gonna be in an IC unit, and you're not gonna die.

Well, sixty-three and a half percent of the people fully vaccinated were dying in England at the exact same time. Why didn't you pull this? Have you ever labeled the President of the United States comment as "misinformation?"

Have you ever done that?

Any of you?

I'll take that as a No.

So again, I'm just wondering who are the authorities— who do you think you are—to censor information from eminently qualified doctors who had the courage and the compassion to treat covid patients when the NIH guideline was basically: If you test positive for covid, go home, be afraid, isolate yourself, don't do anything until you are so sick we'll send you to the hospital, we'll give you Remdesevir, where we have sixteen hundred deaths so far, we'll put you on a vent and we'll watch you die.

You guys bear a fair amount of responsibility for the hundreds of thousands of people not being treated, and I would say probably dying, that didn't have to die. I hope you're proud of yourselves.

Four days later, the CBS news magazine *60 Minutes* featured an interview with President Biden, who declared "The pandemic is over."

Mercifully We Had Answers

Three days after that, attorney Jenin Younes of the New Civil Liberties Alliance, who is representing Dr. Kheriarty and his fellow plaintiffs in *Missouri v Biden*, published a piece in *Tablet* explaining how the government pressure on social media companies crossed over the line from friendly advice to coercion—in other words, censorship.[370] Younes cited numerous examples, such as the previously-mentioned Meta official's obsequious remarks that "it's not great to be accused of killing people" and asserting his desire to "de-escalate and work together collaboratively." Younes noted "These are not the words of a person who is acting freely; to the contrary, they denote the mindset of someone who considers himself subordinate to, and subject to punishment by, a superior."

Younes also discussed the case of *Berenson v Twitter*, in which the former *New York Times* reporter sued the tech giant after he had been removed from that platform. In the process of discovery, Berenson and his lawyers obtained a company memo from an employee who noted that his meeting with a White House official had gone well, even though they had been asked "one really tough question about why Alex Berenson hasn't been kicked off the platform," adding "*mercifully* we had answers." [Emphasis added.] Two months later, after Dr. Fauci had publicly deemed Berenson a danger, and immediately after President Biden's remarks that the social media companies were killing people, Berenson's Twitter account was canceled.

Berenson subsequently won his lawsuit against the tech giant, and his account was reinstated.

Younes noted that the tech giants, many of whom hold monopoly positions, are understandably fearful of incurring the wrath of government bureaucrats—and that anybody in his right mind might well be wary of being held responsible for thousands (or hundreds of thousands) of deaths, and that this chilling effect allowed Drs. Collins, Fauci, and numerous other lesser functionaries to mislead the public into believing there was a scientific consensus on lockdowns, mask mandates, and vaccine mandates.

Younes then goes on to drive her point home:

> The Founders of our country understood that line-drawing becomes virtually impossible once censorship begins and that the personal views and biases of those doing the censoring will inevitably come into play. Moreover, they recognized that sunlight is the best disinfectant: The cure for bad speech is good speech. The cure for lies, truth. Silencing people does not mean problematic ideas disappear; it only drives their adherents into echo chambers.
>
> Indeed, this case could not illustrate more clearly the First Amendment's chief purpose, and why the framers of the Constitution did not create an exception for "misinformation." Government actors are just as prone to bias, hubris, and error as the rest of us. Drs. Fauci and Collins, enamored of newfound fame and basking in self-righteousness, took it

upon themselves to suppress debate about the most important subject of the day. Had Americans learned of the Great Barrington Declaration and been given the opportunity to contemplate its ideas, and had scientists like Bhattacharya, Gupta, and Kulldorff been permitted to speak freely, the history of the pandemic era may have unfolded with far less tragedy—and with far less damage to the institutions that are supposed to protect public health.

Too Big to Fail

Two days after that, I called Dr. Doshi with the question: Where do we go from here? This is what he had to say:

> My sense is that we are dealing with another too-big-to-fail situation. My sense is that this too-big-to-fail situation started in November-December of 2020. And I choose those dates because of two events.
>
> In November, we started to get the press releases about efficacy. The press releases about efficacy, prior to any publication, prior to any data (which we still haven't seen, as you know), that essentially set in motion a desire for the vaccines so strong that only the most hardened toughened critic would have been able to say "Look, I've still got a lot of concerns. There are still a lot of unknowns." And so I think that the situation was very hard for anybody to publicly express a sense of caution. So that's part of what set the too-big-to-fail situation in motion.
>
> And what really, I think, sealed the deal, was the FDA's issuance of the EUA. I argued that the EUA should not have been issued, because the data were far too premature. We didn't have the data on the most important outcomes related

to severe disease, if you're looking at personal protection from infection, if you're thinking about stopping transmission, herd immunity. You can't rush the process. And the process would take time.

And so the only way to thread the needle between balancing the demand that existed with the requirements for more time, if you want credible answers to the important unknown questions about safety and efficacy—the only way to thread that needle was an expanded access program.

Expanded access is used for experimental therapies for people that have, typically, life-threatening conditions who essentially want to try something—anything. And in cases where they can't get into a clinical trial, expanded access says, You can have access to this. There has to be informed consent that the patient understands that we do not know—and can make no assurances—that benefits outweigh risks. And if you're okay with that, then here it is. And it also prohibits any kind of marketing of the product. So you can't charge twenty dollars a dose. You can only charge what it costs to manufacture. That's the most you can charge, if you're charging at all. Typically, manufacturers don't want to release that information—the cost of the manufacturing—so they make it available for free when they do participate in expanded access.

So I thought a large expanded access program—helped by the government—to facilitate the demand where people are saying, you know, "I want it—I'm happy to take the risk." You can imagine this for very high-risk people. A lot of people might be willing to do that. And I thought that was okay. That's the point of expanded access.

But it decouples it from the notion of approval, from the notion of safe and effective, from the notion that everything's been vetted, everything's now clear. And because that didn't happen, and we got an EUA, and the EUA was not treated as it "MIGHT be safe and effective," which is what it's supposed to mean. Instead, it was treated as—and the government promoted it as—"safe and effective." And you could see this. One of the best examples is—not just to refer to our collective memory but a specific instance—is the HHS website—which for months and months used the statutory language "SAFE AND EFFECTIVE" in big bold all-caps lettering—on their home page! That's the statutory standard for, you know, a full approval as we call it these days—a BLA and an NDA.

I never liked the phrase "full approval," by the way, because it suggests there's such a thing as half-approval. It's not a half-approval, right? It's an Emergency Use Authorization. But those events, essentially—the high expectation, and then the sealing of the deal with the EUA which was marketed as "Safe and Effective" and a recommendation was made to go into tens of millions of people.

It is common sense to expect no government could rightly—in their right minds—could ever recommend tens of millions, hundreds of millions of people get a product that they do not have great certainty about the safety and efficacy and the benefits of it. I mean that's just common sense.

At this point, the reader could be forgiven for wondering how Dr. Doshi's proposal for expanded access—with vaccines provided only to those who asked for them, at cost or free of charge—might have been received at the board of directors meeting of Pfizer or Moderna.

People Who Menstruate

The next day, Pfizer CEO Albert Bourla, who had already been double-vaxxed and double-boosted, announced that he had tested positive for covid—for the second time in two months.[371]

Three days after that, the results of an NIH-funded study on the effects of covid vaccines on women's menstrual periods appeared in *BMJ Medicine*.[372] Almost as soon as the vax was made available, such reports had been accumulating, in the scientific literature, in post-marketing reporting systems, and on social media, but this study provided data from a large international cohort, by means of the Natural Cycles digital fertility app.

Why is this important? The paper's authors helpfully explain:

> Although small changes in menstrual characteristics might not be meaningful to clinicians and scientists, any perceived effect to a routine bodily function linked to fertility can be cause for alarm for those experiencing it, and can contribute to vaccine hesitancy. Evan small changes, when unanticipated, can have a large effect on the quality of life of people who menstruate.

The researchers gathered data from 19,622 women across the globe, including 4,686 who had not been vaccinated for the covid and 14,936 who had. Of the latter group, most (nearly eighty-five percent) had taken either the Pfizer or the Moderna shot, while the remainder had received any of a variety of other products, including DNA vaccines (Oxford-AstraZeneca, Janssen, and Sputnik) and traditional killed-virus vaccines (Covaxin, Sinopharm).

They found that the covid vaccines increased the length of a woman's next menstrual cycle by an average of a little less than a day, or almost four days in women who had received both doses in the same cycle—indicating a dose-dependent relationship. The length of the menstrual cycle returned to normal by the second full cycle after vaccination, except for the cohort who had received both doses in the same cycle. There was no observed difference in the effects of the different types of vaccines.

An NIH press release quoted an NIH expert who assured readers "Changes following vaccination appear to be small, within the normal range of variation, and temporary."[373] The press release neglected to mention that previous accounts had included reports of both lengthened and shortened cycles. These opposing effects tend to erase one another when the midpoint of a confidence interval is confused with clinical reality.

The press release also neglected to mention that one out of eight women who received both doses in the same cycle experienced an increase in cycle length of eight days or more—an increase considered by clinicians to be evidence of significant disruption in the functioning of a woman's reproductive system. In addition, they left out any mention of the myriad other reported effects on women's reproductive functioning, including cramps, irregular bleeding, prolonged bleeding, heavier-than-usual bleeding, and breakthrough bleeding in post-menopausal women as well as those on birth control pills or "gender-affirming" hormones.[374] One study found the rate of breakthrough bleeding in post-menopausal women was sixty-six percent.[375] The long-term effects on women's reproductive functioning remain unknown.

While the NIH continues to assure us that all of this is no big deal, not everyone is buying into this ongoing colonization of women's reproductive systems. In her book *The Bodies of Others: The New Authoritarians, COVID-19, and the War against the Human*, author Naomi Wolf wrote:

> All that bleeding, about which I was hearing online and from women I knew, was just not normal. And you didn't have to be a rocket scientist to understand that a dysregulated menstrual cycle was going to negatively affect women's fertility.
>
> It was by listening to women's early anecdotal reports about their own bodies, or about their babies, that we learned

about the dangers of thalidomide and vaginal mesh, silicone breast implants and Mirena.

I am a writer on women's health, and feminism teaches us, "First, listen to women."[376]

Indeed.

CHAPTER FOURTEEN

Listening to Women

The Prof

I caught up with Linda Wastila on one of the last afternoons of the summer of 2022, at Borders Bookstore and Café, just a stone's throw from the Johns Hopkins University Homewood campus. (Disclosure: Linda and I are fellow graduates of the Hopkins Writing Program). We sipped ice teas as she told me about how she and Peter Doshi came up with the idea for the Citizen's Petition:

> The way it happened, both Peter and I were with the University of Maryland System, and on April 23 we got a memorandum from the Chancellor that said everyone had to be vaccinated, and, uh, I kinda freaked out because I wasn't gonna do it. I knew enough at that point that I didn't want it. I have two kids in the system—they're college students. So I reached out to him and I said—we're friends anyways—and I said Let's talk. And he had a random conversation with Kim who he knew with Dave Healy actually, and we came up with the idea of recruiting as many people—scientists, physicians, nationally and internationally—as we could to sign this petition.

On the day that Pfizer was emergency authorized, we got a response from the FDA on our citizen's petition. And it pretty much categorically said every point had no scientific merit.

We were just very upset. I mean, they totally disregarded, totally dismissed everything rolled out. And so we re-trenched. We were exhausted. Putting together the Citizen's Petition was huge. It was so draining. So much time. I was the lead author on it for a couple of reasons. One is because Peter is BMJ Associate Editor, and he didn't want to taint that. And also because he was going up for tenure—and I was safe. You know, I'm tenured.

So we retrenched. [The Citizen's Petition] was so scientific. We needed to pull at heartstrings. So I started harkening back to the AIDS quilts, that sort of thing. Kim is a marketing person. She just—have you ever talked to Kim? Oh God. She's amazing. So we started thinking of a vigil. Then we ended up getting in touch with Bri Dressen, who's running the Survivor's group.

At any rate, we came up with the 11/2 with Senator Johnson round table. Which got absolutely no mainstream press. Not only that, there wasn't a single political representative there. Not a single other one of them, because that's how dangerous it was for us to talk about this, I guess.

So we did that. We've all sort of done our own thing since then. I've been involved in the mandate marches, mostly here in DC. A little bit of background stuff for the LA one. Mostly I'm working now—doing other things behind the scenes. I've worked a lot with the Maryland mandate groups. Done a lot to try to get the system to change those mandates. And the university system. I am a plaintiff on a couple of FOI's and legal suits, including PHMPT. Peter's on that as well.

The Freedom of Information Act request was rejected. FDA said seventy-five years, and then they amended it to ninety-five years and then the judge down in Texas—I forgot who it was—got involved and said No. So we get ten thousand pages a month—the Dump.

Most of it's crap. It's unorganized, there's no table of contents, you have to wade through it.

But we're fighting!

We discussed the matter of Pfizer and Moderna both offering the vax to patients in the placebo arm of the trial, long before the trial was slated to end—in effect eliminating the control group:

> If they can get rid of the control group, then we don't know what's going on. We don't know what's normative. And when they have these clinical trials, they're supposed to go on to 2023, 2024, some of them even longer term. But if you don't have a control group, how can you do it? I mean, what are you going to present? Six months is not long for efficacy. Certainly we do have the studies that have shown that your antibody response drops precipitously after about three months.

The issue of waning immunity led quite naturally to a discussion of the potential problems with repeated booster shots. Dr. Wastila had this to say:

> Essentially what you are doing with repeated exposure is you are priming your B-cells and T-cells to be hyper-reactive. So your body is creating more spike protein. More responses to everything. You get hyper-immune. Which makes it more likely to suffer other adverse consequences, more susceptible to chronic diseases like autoimmune things.

Like MS. Like lupus. All this fatigue and tiredness. There's POTS. This stuff is all autoimmune-related. It's kicking crap up that's in your body right now. It's probably been handled well by your healthy immune system prior to this, and now it's wreaking havoc.

I think that's why people are—I don't know how many people you know who have Stage Four cancer, but you know something? I know five—six! I just thought of someone else. Three in my writing group—two are dead. Dead. Dead. Cancer out of nowhere. And that's part of that response. That's part of that response.

We talked about long covid (which Dr. Wastila says she herself suffered from), vaccine reactogenicity, and the difficulties of distinguishing between the two. Dr. Wastila summed up matters thusly:

I sympathize with everybody except for the people who are trying to push this shit on me and on my kids. It's horrible. It's the biggest medical scandal ever.

That's quite a statement. Do you care to explain what you mean by that?

We've had more people exposed to this product in a short period of time using a novel technology which we know nothing about other than they've tried to do it for decades for the common cold. And then covid came. It's miraculously here. There's patents for this platform for the coronavirus. There's actually discussions about how to treat a novel coronavirus before the coronavirus actually came.

And the levels of the monies that went in to mandate use, to coerce the use, the executive orders that went in, the briberies that went in, especially to young people, is unprecedented. And the number of people who are dying, have complications, from this product, from these products, is already way beyond the number of people who had actually succumbed to covid. Of course, most of them succumbed with covid, not from covid. And there's no liability for the producer. So there's no recourse.

We are essentially maiming and killing—in my opinion, it's going to be millions before this is over. I really believe it. The excess mortality records that are coming out of life insurers now—and you know they're going to be bailed out, and it'll be hush-hush—the data will disappear.

I know I sound like a conspiracy theorist, but I look at data. I look at data all the time. That's my job. And these data are legit. I mean, excess mortality in young people—as I said, in my social circle in the last six months—I know six people who have Stage Four cancers that were either totally in remission and had been for years and decades, or it came out of nowhere and it was symptomless and they were dead.

Mindful of the fact that just the night before, President Biden had declared "the pandemic is over," I asked Dr. Wastila if she concurred:

My opinion is that the mRNA platform is the future of almost all medications. In general the pharmaceutical industry has not had a good pipeline. They didn't have a lot in the pipeline. And then covid came along.

And for whatever reason—this mRNA platform—why it was all of a sudden ready to go—I've got my suspicions on that. And now they're talking about using it for every vaccine. They're talking about using it more for cancer, where most of the work has been. They're talking about using it for all sorts of applications as a platform.

So covid itself may be—it might be over—but what the pandemic did, and what this disease did—the technologies in terms of the vaccines, the mRNA technology—it provided the launching ground for the future of pharmaceuticals. And I don't think it's gonna be a pretty future.

Towards the end of our conversation, Dr. Wastila asks me whom else I plan to interview for the book. I reel off a list of names, most of whom she says she knows well, and this segues into a bit of self-reflection, on how her campaign has affected her personally:

I'm in a new world. I've lost all my other friends for the most part. Because I've been so outspoken about this stuff I became a bit of a pariah in my own school. These are my new friends. My tribe.

The Whistleblower

When I went into this, I was just shocked. I mean, I had no idea.

So says Brook Jackson, former clinical trial auditor for Ventavia Research Group and current plaintiff in the False Claims Act lawsuit against Pfizer.

I've spent twenty years helping bring therapeutics, biologics, devices to the market. I'm not anti-vax. I'm not anti-government. I felt proud to work on this trial.

In September of 2020, Brook went to work for Ventavia, owner of three of the 153 sites which carried out the trials which served as the basis for FDA approval of the Pfizer shot. She was appalled by what she saw:

It was nothing like anything I've ever been a part of. They just had no regard for patients at all.

They were severely understaffed. For Pfizer specifically, they had five coordinators when we needed triple that number. They were getting so many phone calls and diary entries of adverse events that they just could not keep up. The voice mailboxes were full. Patients were eventually having to reach out directly to Pfizer.

Brook told me that the tasks of assessing eligibility and performing physicals were carried out not by doctors or nurses but by "research coordinators," who are not licensed to practice medicine, and then the investigator would just sign off on the source documents. Two of these coordinators were medical assistants, and a third was a former restaurant cashier who doubled as the receptionist for Ventavia. This person (with no medical training whatsoever) had been entrusted with preparing doses of the Pfizer product, administering injections, and assessing patients post-injection for complications. Brook also told me that during the eighteen days she spent working for Ventavia, she met the "Principal Investigator" exactly once, and she never met any of the designated "sub-investigators" at all.

In her role as trial auditor, Brook checked the clinic's crash cart, which contains materials to be used to treat patients in cases of emergency. The norepinephrine was missing, and the Benadryl had expired. Both of these medications are used to treat cases of severe allergic reaction—a rare but potentially life-threatening complication of vaccines.

Blood samples were routinely mislabeled by overworked staffers—so many that Pfizer complained that multiple specimens had the same bar code. Symptomatic patients were not tested for COVID-19 because of a lack of supplies.

One day Brook checked the biohazard bags and found they contained used needles—a blatant violation of basic safety protocols. (Used needles are to be disposed of in a sharps container.) She describes what happened next:

So I walk around to the reception area and I see the whiteboard had post-it notes with patients' full names, addresses, social security numbers, W-9 forms the patients had completed. I was shocked. Health information wasn't protected at all. Anyone could walk through there and see exactly what I was seeing.

I ask Brook if she communicated her concerns to her superiors:

Yes. Every single day. Starting from Day One. Wow. I was bringing my concerns to our 8:00 AM call that we held every morning.

At first they seemed sympathetic to her concerns, but about halfway through her time there they changed their tune:

At this point it goes from Let's make these changes, let's do training, let's get life support, let's hire more qualified people, let's get registered nurses, let's bring in more investigators who have the time to devote to clinical research.

So it went from that to Brook, we know we have a problem, but the goal right now is to continue to do what Pfizer wants us to do, and that's enroll more patients.

Brook discovered that Ventavia had printed forms denoting treatment group assignments for each patient. These forms were inserted into every patient's chart—a blatant violation of the fundamental principle of a double-blind trial, which is that neither patients nor clinicians should know who is getting the active drug and who is getting placebo. According to Pfizer's own protocols, these data never should have been used. Instead, Ventavia removed the forms from the patients' charts and had them shredded.

Brook tried contacting Pfizer (after hours, using a phone number not linked to her) but she was unable to speak to a live human being. So she communicated her concerns in an email to the FDA, and six hours later she was fired.

Brook hired an attorney, initially with the intention of filing a wrongful termination suit against Ventavia, but the more she went over her experience there the more she felt she had grounds for a False Claims Act case.

After meeting with twenty-five or more attorneys, she finally chose one to represent her in her lawsuit. After taking sixty days to investigate, the federal government decided it needed an additional six months to look into the matter. In the meantime, the vax was rolled out, not just to high-risk patients but to everyone—adolescents, children, pregnant women—and millions were coerced into taking the shot on pain of losing their jobs. The FDA inspected six of 153 Pfizer trial sites. Ventavia was not included. And all this time, Brook was under a gag order.

Then in September, the FDA requested another six-month extension:

> And I thought, they're never gonna do anything. They're going to get this vaccine into as many arms as they can. They're just gonna keep requesting extension after extension and never do a damn thing about inspecting and investigating my allegations. And people are dying and people are being hurt by this product. And so in September, I said to my attorneys that I wasn't gonna be quiet anymore.

Brook appeared on *Tucker Carlson Tonight* and told her story. Two days later her attorneys fired her. One told her in an email "If you go public with your story, the government is going to come after you."

Brook reached out to Dr. Doshi, who put her in touch with Paul Thacker, the *BMJ* investigative journalist who covered her story, and also obtained new legal representation. Her story broke on 2 November 2021—the same day the meeting of the Expert Panel on Federal Vaccine Mandates was convened by Senator Johnson. Brook attended the meeting:

Sitting there and listening to these people share their experiences, every one of these stories, they've just touched me so much. And now the focus has kind of changed.

For me, it's really about giving a voice to those who have been injured by this and that is why I cannot stop fighting now.

I ask Brook if she expects to be deposed by Pfizer's lawyers. She smiles confidently and replies "I hope so."

The Advocate

Annapolis, mid-October, mid-morning. I'm sitting across the table from Jenin Younes, litigation counsel for the New Civil Liberties Alliance, in the shade behind the Starbucks on West Street. It's really a bit too chilly for outdoor seating at this point but neither of us notices, focused as we are on the matters at hand—*Missouri v Biden* and AB 2098, which had been signed into law three weeks earlier by California Governor Gavin Newsom.

I begin our conversation by playing the Devil's advocate. In regard to *Missouri v Biden*, I point out that nobody at the tech companies has been imprisoned, nobody has been fined, nobody has been charged, nobody has been arrested, nobody has lost his job. "So in what sense is this coercion?" I ask.

Well, Biden and members of the administration have threatened regulatory action. You know, Section 230 [of the Communications Decency Act] currently protects the tech companies from liability for what people say on their platforms. They've made statements about the tech companies possibly being held accountable for people's deaths from covid. I don't know what the legal theory for doing that would be, but I suppose someone could come up with something. Nobody wants to be sued for killing people. Even if the lawsuit wasn't ultimately successful.

So it's not entirely clear, but the administration certainly has the authority to do some of these things, and they've also acted outside the bounds of their authority. The fact that they're making threats to do something would reasonably scare companies.

I then query her about AB 2098, the bill criminalizing the spreading of "false information" regarding covid treatments and vaccines by doctors. Again playing the Devil's advocate, I point out that doctors have always been enjoined from malpractice, which presumably would include giving patients false or misleading information. "What's new about this bill?" I inquire.

The biggest problem is that it defines false or misleading information as anything that deviates from the scientific consensus. That's absurd. I mean, who gets to define what scientific consensus is? And when you're censoring people, there might be an apparent consensus that isn't the actual consensus. So you actually have the government deciding what the truth is, which is very disturbing.

Doctors are supposed to rely on their own judgment, their own research. And they're not supposed to all have uniform decisions. That's one reason you pick your doctor, because you like their approach.

Younes mentions the case of a doctor who treated severe appendicitis with antibiotics rather than surgery, and had survival rates that surpassed those of his professional colleagues:

The so-called consensus was behind him. It took ten years before that became a standard practice. The idea that we're gonna hamstring doctors—how can we know? He was using his own experience to make judgements, and that's what professionals are supposed to do.

Younes goes on to point out that traditionally, cases of malpractice have always had to involve evidence of identifiable harm to a specific individual. Under AB 2098, this no longer is the case. A doctor could be sanctioned (for example) for telling a patient that masks don't work.

The conversation turns to more general matters. I ask her, Why do you do what you do?

> I'm terrified by the way that governments have corrupted the science to suit the interests of the pharmaceutical companies.
>
> These are the most important civil rights issues of our time.

Younes goes on to express her concerns regarding the erosion of trust in public institutions created by mandates and pandemic restrictions:

> I think that by constantly lying to the American public—the CDC and other agencies and public health authorities—a lot of Americans simply don't trust them anymore. I don't trust them at all.
>
> That's one of the reasons I got into the litigation. Because I had been talking to Drs. Kulldorff and Bhattacharya, and they were saying That's not how you do public health. You use persuasion, you give people the facts, you let them make their own decisions. That's how you build trust—not by censoring and lying. We know the CDC and other agencies have lied. They've lied about the evidence that that vaccine stops transmission. They've lied about the efficacy of masks. And nobody trusts them anymore. And that's a problem. You want to have institutions you can trust.

I think they think people are stupid. They think, We know what's best for them. It's okay if we lie to them. They think we are stupid sheep.

The Scientist

We have seen a rise in infections with RSV as well as flu in children as well as in older adults. And living in a bubble never helps. The fact is that we have lived in a bubble since "shelter-in-place" was first announced in March 2020, and we are paying the price for it.

So says Aditi Bhargava, a molecular and cell biologist and Professor Emeritus in the Biomedical Sciences Graduate Program at the University of California San Francisco, when asked about the skyrocketing rates of respiratory infections following two and a half years of lockdowns, school closures, anti-social distancing, and the like.

I ask Dr. Bhargava about the waning of immunity induced by the mRNA vaccines. "Why does the immunity fade? Does anybody have a guess?"

She laughs and replies "I don't think we need to guess."

We know that vaccine-induced immunity is never, never lifelong. It's not been lifelong even for the best of vaccines. If you look at smallpox or chicken pox vaccines, their effectiveness in a real world scenario is pretty high—over eighty percent. And even that immunity goes away in five to seven years. So it's not like developing life-long immunity after a natural infection with these childhood diseases.

So for the infectious diseases such as smallpox and chicken pox, when you get them as a child, then your immune system has the potential to train itself to develop life-long immunity. And that training is very different than when you get infected with seasonal viruses such as influenza, or corona. Those give you, not lifelong, but multiple years of immunity.

There has been a study done by Imperial College of London that showed that people who got the flu in the years prior to 2019, who were not vaccinated [against COVID-19], they did not get covid, despite being exposed. So you get this kind of cross protection from natural infection of related viruses.

Vaccine is sort of like giving you a shortcut. In traditional vaccines, they take a dead or attenuated virus and give you that. And that, to a large extent, overlaps and mimics a natural infection.

But that's not the case with the mRNA vaccines. If you compare people who got naturally infected with covid and were not vaccinated, the kind of immune response you see in them is much wider and more polyclonal, with early IgA neutralizing antibody response, and the spike antibody component has far less contribution. Whereas in vaccine-induced immunity, the spike protein is the only component to which antibodies can be made.

You're giving only a small portion of the virus, and you are forcing your body to make antibodies only to a small portion of the virus.

In a natural infection, most of the neutralizing antibodies are not the kind of antibodies that the mRNA vaccines are making.

So it's assumed that these vaccines are providing you protection or reducing symptoms or reducing hospitalizations. There is no systematic study that's been done to show that.

We talk about Dr. Bhargava's People's Response to Vaccine Efficacy and Safety (PROVES) Study, and what she and her colleagues have learned about the effects of the vax on women's reproductive health:

> We have data from over ten thousand people. And our study is different from the other studies which have reported changes in the menstrual cycle after getting the mRNA vaccine. Most of those studies don't have a good control population. Ideally, we should use each person as their own control—before the vaccine, what was happening to them versus after the vaccine. Right?
>
> We find quite a high percentage of women reporting irregularities in their menstrual cycle after getting the covid vaccine.
>
> It's extremely concerning, because we just don't understand what the long-term effects are going to be. Whether or not it affects their ability to have children later on—who knows? And if that's the case, you know, if they haven't had children before, they'll just say their infertility is of unknown etiology. If scientists and medical professionals are having problem acknowledging that these vaccines have adverse events, how will they ever acknowledge that this could be ever a contributing factor to infertility?

Her mention of control groups prompts me to ask "Why do you think they have been so eager to get people who have already recovered from the covid to get the shot?"

> I think it's a great way to fudge the data. If you give the vaccine to everybody, irrespective of whether they have had covid or not, whether they are otherwise healthy or immunocompromised, then we don't have a good case-control study.

And for no other vaccine is this ever done—vaccinating people who have recovered from natural infection. This goes against the basic tenets of immunology. You go back and read the literature before 2020, everywhere, whoever was designing vaccines, their main goal was to be able to mimic natural immunity, So why is suddenly natural immunity not good enough, and just for covid?

Dr. Bhargava points out that we have had coronavirus epidemics before—SARS-CoV-1 and MERS-CoV, and that every time the pandemic was gone before a vaccine could be deployed:

> So this time they had to make sure they were able to get the vaccine in people before the epidemic was gone, because now they've spent billions and billions of dollars developing these vaccines for decades. So just because billions of dollars have been spent, they need to recover the money
>
> Just like the banks were too big to fail, this enterprise has become too big to fail.
>
> People's health is collateral damage in this war against covid.

The Mom

> I hiked and climbed and skied and snowboarded and went camping and did all the outdoor things. My kids were skiing as soon as they could. Our house was a revolving door of people from our communities, kids, families. It was a good time.

That's how Brianne Dressen remembers her life—before she volunteered as a human subject for the Oxford-AstraZeneca COVID-19 vaccine trial.

Since then, her life has changed in ways she scarcely could have imagined. We met via Zoom, as she lay on her left side in bed, covered by two fleece blankets, propped up by two pillows.

Brianne, who hails from Salt Lake City, is married with two small children. Her husband is a research chemist, while Bri ran her own preschool. They both shared a deep sense of obligation to serve their community, to help those less fortunate than themselves. They volunteered at the Ronald McDonald House, making lunches and dinner for the families of sick children. They collected toys for foster kids and children in detention homes. They made kits for homeless people, providing them with gift cards, socks, and toothbrushes.

Bri explains:

> Our kids had everything that they could need. They had a stable, loving home with dual income parents that were educated. And so we wanted them to see that life isn't actually that way for much of society. And so we wanted to give them the opportunity to see these other parts of society that needed us to help them.

When the pandemic started, Bri made face masks to donate to the community, and when she had the opportunity to volunteer for the vaccine trial, it seemed like the natural thing to do—another chance to serve.

Before she got the first shot of what was intended to be a two-dose series, Bri had to sign a disclosure agreement that was more than twenty pages long, initialing each page along with adding the date and time:

> And in the contract, one of the things there was auto-antibody enhancement with chimpanzees and they were like, But we don't know if this will happen with humans, so don't worry about it. So it's like, Okay, that's weird. And then the other thing was they promised to pay any and all expenses as a result of injury, which they didn't do.

And another thing in the contract was that they're gonna follow everybody for two years.

They also signed her up for the company's tracking app, which could register only adverse events pre-selected by the company.

Bri received her first dose of the vax. Within an hour things began going wrong:

> I had a tingling down the same arm into my hand. And that one was just on the ride home from the clinic. So it was within the first hour that my issues started. Later than night after dinner my vision became blurry and double.
>
> And then around that same time sound became distorted. It sounded like I had tin cans over my ears.

The next morning she was limping. She felt acutely sensitive to sound and light, and that day at preschool she parked her young charges in front of a learning channel and repeatedly implored them to lower their voices.

That day was her last day as a preschool teacher.

Bri and her husband called every neurology clinic in town. None of them could see her, but when they heard her recitation of symptoms they advised her to go to the emergency room, which she did—only to be diagnosed with anxiety.

Bri returned to the ER several times after that, for irregular heartbeat. Each time she was again diagnosed with anxiety and prescribed benzos or antidepressants:

> I still had a fever. I had a fever literally for months. My vision was messed up for months. My hearing was messed up for months. The pins and needles and electrical sensations, I still have those to this day.
>
> I started having diarrhea. I lost twenty pounds in two months because everything just went straight through me.

Let's see—what else happened? Oh, severe rashes. The tremors, which we learned are actually adrenaline dumps.

I remember shaking uncontrollably on the floor and my kids came over and they were like What's wrong, Mom? And I was like, It's fine, it's fine. And they were like Oh, she must be cold. And so they put a blanket on me haphazardly and then they ran off and played.

My kids were used to me engaging in all their activities and playing with them and doing everything. So my little girl would come and be like, Mom, color with me. And I remember I was just laying there shaking, and she just put her coloring book down on the floor next to me and just started coloring while I was shaking uncontrollably, and then inside I'm like, I hope I don't die here in front of my kid.

I ended up in the ER with heart rate fluctuations. My heart rate skyrocketed up to two hundred and twenty. Before this, I was athletic, my heart rate was in the forties and fifties.

I could hardly breathe. It felt like someone was sitting on my chest all the time.

Her muscles wasted away, and she became incontinent. She suffered severe tinnitus, with a roaring sound in one ear and a high-pitched whine in the other.

Bri was admitted to hospital, where she was diagnosed with "anxiety due to the covid vaccine." She was sent home with instructions for in-home physical therapy and occupational therapy, and she set off on the path to recovery, exercising the same determination she had in every other area of her life:

There was no point where I was going to be the person who was going to lay in bed. I was gonna be up and trying to figure out how to get my nerves all talking to each other again. Every day I was gonna get up and fix this.

My husband helped me walk every day. It was get up and move, get up and move, get up and move. So even when my legs weren't working, I still was getting my husband to prop me up on my spin bike. And I was trying to push down with my knees to just try to get my legs to move right again.

My husband took me outside one day. We live on a hill, and I remember my feet landing on the driveway that's on a slant and it felt like it was the first time I had ever touched uneven ground in my life. Everything was brand new again. And so I had to learn to walk on uneven ground again. I had to learn to go up and down the stairs again. I was determined I was going to get every part of my body talking together again.

But at the same time I was also having cognitive problems. My memory was shot. My personality just completely shifted. I didn't have the connection I had with my kids anymore.

My skin felt like it was on fire. I was flat inside, emotionally just flat and dead.

Her sister, a doctor, observed "It's like the vaccine gave you autism." Bri had thoughts of ending it all:

The only reason I'm alive is because my husband did not leave me alone for one minute while I was in that situation. And it's not like that went on for hours or days. I was in that place in my head for months.

Unsurprisingly, the clinical research organization where Bri received her first shot advised her not to get the second one:

In the clinical trial report, they say that people elected to
forego the second shot for unexplained reasons, which is total
BS. They tracked me for about two months, and then they
stopped tracking my data.

The clinical trial company would call and say, Hey, do
you have any updates? And usually on those calls I would be
crying, right?

Cause I'd be like, Please can you guys help me? Has
AstraZeneca called you back? And they're like, No, Astra-
Zeneca hasn't called us. What's going on? And then I just
tell them through the tears, I'm still not working. I still can't
use my legs. I still can't eat, I still can't sleep. All I can do is
breathe.

And that's how it was. It was horrible. Worst experience
in my life, by far. Terrifying. Nobody knew what was going
on, nobody had answers, and nobody was gonna help.

Bri's husband and sister procured the services of a local doctor who
was able to give her the assistance she needed:

Over the span of the next eight, nine months we trialed a ton
of meds. Literally tens of thousands of dollars' worth of meds
to figure out what was going to tamp down on things. So I
didn't feel like I was dying all the time.

So it calmed my heart. So my palpitations calmed down,
my tachycardia calmed down, my chest pain slowly went
away. I had to re-train my diaphragm to breathe correctly.

Bri's husband reached out to doctors and researchers all over the world,
trying to find the cause of her torment. He asked a German laboratory to
analyze a blood sample, and they found anti-neuronal auto-antibodies—a
contingency the disclosure agreement had warned about. After trying
(and failing) to get local doctors and hospitals to administer Intravenous

Immunoglobulin (IVIG) therapy, he reached out to the National Institutes of Health. In June of 2021, Bri was flown out to the NIH where she finally received a diagnosis of vaccine injury and began receiving IVIG for her woes.

She continues to receive the treatment, at a cost of some eleven hundred dollars (slated to go up to sixteen hundred dollars in January), twice a month. But the family now has to get by on one income, and they have had to hire a nanny to care for the children. In order to pay for the IVIG and a myriad of other treatments, they have burned through their retirement savings, and re-mortgaged their home.

The drugmaker offered the family $590 for their expenses. When they refused, they upped the offer to twelve hundred dollars, in exchange for them signing a waiver exempting the company from any further liability. Needless to say, the offer was spurned.

Upon her return from the NIH, Bri, insofar as her health allowed her to, began reaching out to other sufferers of covid vaccine injuries. Together, they founded React19, a patient advocacy organization. They reached out to the NIH, the CDC, the FDA. None of these agencies were interested in helping. They reached out to their elected representatives—Democrats first, then Republicans. ("To be honest, most of us that were injured were Democrats," she explains.) None of them were interested in helping either, except for the one man who went on to champion their cause—Wisconsin Senator Ron Johnson.

Bri tells me many of fellow vaccine injury sufferers have endured so much pain, with no end in sight, that they have contemplated suicide:

> So we have to tell people, Look, you have to live for other people, sadly cause that'll just destroy them. And that's pulled me out of my place many, many, many times. Like, that is not an option. I have to exist this way. That's not an option cause it would destroy my family, destroy 'em for the rest of their lives. So it's better for me to exist like this and to suffer every

single day, than it is for me to choose to end that suffering, because it would destroy them.

All this talk of family prompts me to ask, What does being a mother mean to you? This is what she has to say:

> It's everything. So being able to take care of my kids and be their mom was the most important thing in the world to me. And then to have that stripped from me—now my kids take care of me, instead of me taking care of them—that's been one of the worst punishments of this whole thing.
>
> Of all the titles I've had in my life, Mom has been the most significant and the one that I'm the most proud of.

The Widow

> He was super funny. He's always been super funny.

That's how Kim Witczak remembers her late husband, Woody.

It has been a long journey for Kim, beginning with the untimely demise of a loved one, her search for answers, her lawsuit against Pfizer which revealed how the company had concealed the harms caused by its product, and her years of service on FDA committees as consumer representative, all of which led to her current focus on uncovering the truth about the Pfizer shots.

This is someone whom the FDA listens to, and this is someone who knows what Pfizer is capable of. Her journey began nearly two decades ago, after the life two young people had planned together was shattered by a prescription for Pfizer's blockbuster drug Zoloft.

Woody had been her first boyfriend. Her one and only. Kim met Woody one evening at a bar where she was celebrating her birthday with her friends. They ended up sitting together on the sidewalk and talking until 3:00 AM. They were inseparable after that, and three years later they got married.

> He was loud. He'd walk into a room and you felt his energy.
> He was smart, well read. He would challenge things—
> sometimes to the point where it would drive me a little crazy.
> I remember sometimes if we were out with our friends and
> he'd start saying something, I'd kick him under the table, and
> then he'd be like "Why are you kicking me?" And I was like,
> "Okay, you're such an ass."

Woody was a sharp dresser, meticulously organized, and meticulous about his health. He never had more than one drink in the course of an evening. Both Woody and Kim would arise at 6:00 AM to work out together. At the time of his demise, Woody had been training to run his first marathon.

Both were successful professionals—he was employed in sales, she in advertising. Although both worked full-time, they lived on just one income. They were determined to chart their own course, and not be slaves to debt.

Although both had jobs that required extensive travel, they stayed in touch even when apart. They would leave notes in each other's suitcases, and talk on the phone several times a day.

> He took good care of me. He took good, good care of me.

In 2003, Woody landed his dream job at a start-up and, in the excitement, was having trouble sleeping. He went to his trusted primary care doctor, who prescribed medication for his condition. Meanwhile, Kim was away for a photo shoot for a client in New Zealand. The assignment required her to be out of the country for three weeks.

When Kim returned home, she knew right away something was wrong. Woody looked haggard—thinner, perhaps. He was drenched in sweat, curled up on the kitchen floor, rocking back and forth, groaning "You gotta help me. My head's outside my body, looking in."

> Obviously I had never seen this behavior before from him. I remember trying to calm him down. Let's pray, let's breathe.
>
> He called the doctor and told him what happened. The doctor said you gotta give the drug four to six weeks to kick in.

Nobody suspected the drug could be the cause of all this.

On their last Saturday together, Kim and Woody hosted an engagement party for two of their friends. Woody proudly showed off their house to the guests. He seemed back to normal. But the next day he confided to Kim that he had been suffering nightmares—visions so terrifying he could not bring himself to describe them to her.

The next day Kim left for Detroit for a four-day photo shoot. They had big plans for her return. For their tenth anniversary, they planned to visit Thailand, and after that they intended to have children and start a family, at last.

But none of this ever came to be.

Kim departed on Monday morning. That following evening she called Woody, and they spoke for a long time, as was their custom.

The next day, Kim went to work. Woody didn't call, as he normally would have done. Kim telephoned Woody's mother and asked if she had heard from him. She hadn't. She checked their voice mail. There was a call from one of Woody's business partners, reminding him of an important meeting scheduled for the next day, and asking why he hadn't checked in.

Kim called her father and asked him to check on Woody. He called her back with these stark words: "It's bad."

What do you mean It's bad? And he's like, he's dead. How do you know he's dead? He's hanging.

Woody hadn't even left a suicide note.

Kim put down the phone and screamed. One of her co-workers took her back to the hotel where she was staying.

> I remember the coroner called and asked if Woody was on any medication. I'm like, I don't know, there's something that's upstairs in our medicine cabinet.
>
> She goes, there's a bottle of Zoloft siting on the kitchen counter. We're gonna take it with us. It might have something to do with his death.

By an odd coincidence, that same day the local newspaper ran an article noting that drug regulators in the UK had found a link between antidepressants and suicide.

Kim's brother-in-law Eric—her sister's husband—knew something had gone terribly wrong. Woody hadn't been suicidal—indeed, he was a man who had everything to live for.

Eric googled "Zoloft and suicide." He pored over every book he could find on the subject—including *The Antidepressant Fact Book* by Peter Breggin and *Let Them Eat Prozac* by David Healy.

After the funeral, Kim found herself in the basement of their home, gazing at a photograph of her late husband.

> I kept crying God, take my pain away and use it.

The next night Eric came over and told her "I think I figured out what happened to Woody."

And that is how Kim became, in her own words, "the accidental advocate." The following year she and Dr. Healy met with FDA officials, one of whom told Kim her husband's death was "an anecdote."

Kim filed a wrongful death suit against Pfizer. The corporate behemoth deposed family and friends and neighbors, trying to find something—anything—to pin Woody's death on besides Zoloft.

They deposed Kim as well, insinuating that she had been having an extramarital affair with Woody's business partner, and even inquiring about Woody's habit of sweeping the driveway every morning—as if this were somehow evidence of mental illness.

In the course of discovery, Kim's lawyers obtained documents proving patients in Pfizer's trials of Zoloft had reported they felt they were standing outside their bodies—exactly as Woody had before his death.

Pfizer knew.

After the suit had been settled, Kim continued her advocacy work, eventually landing a spot on the FDA Psychopharmacologic Drug Advisory Committee. But when Pfizer appealed for the black box warning on Chantix to be lifted, Kim was removed from the panel by the agency, which cited her "intellectual bias."

Undaunted, Kim flew to Washington DC at her own expense and testified before the panel as a private citizen, imploring them not to lift the warning while the evidence from well over two thousand cases that had been settled by Pfizer remained under lock and key.

All of these words of caution fell upon deaf ears.

How has this campaign affected her personally? Kim pauses for a moment of self-reflection:

> I've always been told "You're so strong. You don't ever get emotional." And I say "You just don't see me behind closed doors. You don't see me when I go home to an empty house."

Kim's advocacy work continues. Her current focus on the mRNA shots, she explains, is a natural outgrowth of her work on Pfizer's blockbuster drug Zoloft and other SSRI's. She points out that Pfizer, which had never made vaccines, has been granted complete legal immunity for damages inflicted by its product. She also mentions that the Pfizer trial, which was supposed to go on for two years, was stopped after just a small fraction of participants had made it to the six-month mark. At that point all participants were offered the shot, in effect eliminating the control group.

"That means the real world is going to be the actual clinical trial," she tells me.

We have already recounted her testimony before VRBPAC urging the FDA to hold off on emergency use authorization of the Pfizer shot, along with her roles in the Citizen's Petition, the lawsuit which forced the Pfizer Data Dump, and the meeting of the Expert Panel convened by Senator Ron Johnson on 2 November 2021.

Kim testified at the meeting of the Expert Panel, and afterwards she posted a video of her testimony on Vimeo—which, she tells me, was promptly removed.

She goes on to discuss meeting Brianne Dressen, Maddie de Garay, Ernest Ramirez, and others who took the shot (or whose loved ones took the shot) in good faith, as prescribed, and suffered devastating consequences.

They're being gaslit—told it's all in their head.

Just like Kim and Woody.

The conversation turns to other matters. I ask Kim, What kind of father do you think Woody would have made?

> He would have been an amazing dad. I know the way he was with his nieces. He never missed a birthday party. He would fly down there for their birthday parties. He would always stay an extra day to go to their baseball game or their basketball games.
>
> He always said, I will never judge my life based on how much money I make, or my career. It'll be based on my family and friends and leaving the world a better place. And we just

never got that chance of the legacy of kids. So I wanted to give him another kind of legacy.

I then ask her what kind of mother she thinks she would have made. She doesn't hesitate before replying:

I think I would have made a great mom.

CHAPTER FIFTEEN

For the Good of Society

October–November 2022

Less Than Zero

On the first day of October, a study released in preprint form by University of Maryland researchers reported that the efficacy of the Moderna product in preventing infection by the Omicron variant dropped to less than zero five months after the booster shot.[377]

The study was funded by Moderna.

Six days later, Florida Surgeon General Joseph Ladapo formally recommended against COVID-19 mRNA vaccines for males ages eighteen through thirty-nine: "With a high level of global immunity to COVID-19, the benefit of vaccination is likely outweighed by this abnormally high risk of cardiac-related death among men in this age group."[378] The press release also contained these words:

> The Department continues to stand by its Guidance for Pediatric COVID-19 vaccines issued in March 2022, which recommends against use in healthy children and adolescents 5 years old to 17 years old. This now includes recommendations against COVID-19 vaccination among infants and

children under 5 years old, which has since been issued under Emergency Use Authorization.

Once again Dr. Gorski joined in the fray:

> This is the first time that we've seen a state government weaponize bad science to spread antivaccine disinformation as official policy, a dangerous new escalation in antivaccine propaganda.[379]

The following Monday, Janine Small, President of International Developed Markets for Pfizer, was testifying before the European Union Parliament when the following exchange took place:[380]

> Q: Was the Pfizer Covid Vaccine tested on stopping the transmission of the virus before it entered the market? If not, please say it clearly. If yes, are you willing to share the data with this committee? And I really want a straight answer, yes or no, and I'm looking forward to it.

> A: Regarding the question around, um, did we know about stopping the immunisation [sic] before it entered the market? No.

Small was giggling nervously as she delivered her answer. She went on to add:

> Um, these, um, you know, we really had to move at the speed of science to really understand what is taking place in the market, and from that point of view we had to do everything at risk. I think Dr Bourla, even though he's not here, would turn around and say to you himself, "If not us then who?"

The fact that the vax was authorized for emergency use without any data purporting to show it reduced transmission was not news—the FDA had made this clear way back in December of 2020—but Small's testimony brought this matter to the public's attention in a way that could not be ignored.

Again the fact-checkers swung into play. After acknowledging that every single detail in the story was correct, a piece by RMIT FactLab quoted Julie Leask, "a social scientist who specializes in immunisation," who averred that the story "heavily distorts the facts," and also indirectly quoted a Pfizer spokesperson who noted the trial was designed and powered to test the vaccine's efficacy on preventing "disease and severe disease."[381]

Now strictly speaking, this was true—obviously severe cases are included in the total number of cases—but it was a spectacularly disingenuous way of spinning the truth (which had been openly acknowledged all along) that the trial was not powered to measure the effect on severe cases *as a separate endpoint*.

Were the "fact-checkers" themselves guilty of "heavily distorting the facts?"

Three days later, the Supreme Court of the State of New York ordered all New York City employees who had been fired for refusing the shot be re-hired with back pay. The court's decision reiterated a key point which by now was obvious to all—that the shot did not stop infection or transmission.

On 18 October Moderna CEO Stéphane Bancel stated that the covid boosters should be reserved only for people over the age of fifty and those with underlying health conditions—in direct contradiction to the CDC recommendation that everyone over the age of five should get vaccinated.[382]

And yet, just two days after that, the CDC voted to approve adding the covid shots to the childhood vaccine schedule.[383] Two days after that, the CDC announced that Director Rochelle Walensky, who already had been double-vaxxed and triple boosted, had come down with the covid.[384]

On the last day of the month, an article appeared in the *Atlantic* titled "The Worst Pediatric-Care Crisis in Decades."[385] Author Katherine J. Wu, a PhD microbiologist from Harvard, painted a grim picture of pediatric intensive-care units overwhelmed with toddlers and children suffering from a miscellany of respiratory infections, including influenza, rhinovirus, enterovirus, and respiratory syncytial virus.

The culprit? In Dr. Wu's own words:

> With the pandemic's great viral vanishing, kids missed out on early encounters that would have trained up their bodies' defensive cavalry.

In plain English: More than two years of lockdowns, school closures, anti-social distancing, and being slathered with hand sanitizer meant that the little ones had been deprived of the antigenic challenges needed to build healthy immune functioning, and now they are sitting ducks for a whole mélange of respiratory infections.

This is precisely the scenario covid skeptics had been warning us about for almost three years.

A Hefty Element of Luck

That same day, another article appeared in the *Atlantic*, this one by Brown University Economics Professor Emily Oster—whom, as you may recall, had called for covid vaccine refusers to be fired from their jobs the previous December. Titled "Let's Declare a Pandemic Amnesty,"[386] the piece contained these words of wisdom:

> Obviously some people intended to mislead and made wildly irresponsible claims. Remember when the public-health community had to spend a lot of time and resources urging Americans not to inject themselves with bleach? That was bad. Misinformation was, and remains, a huge problem. But most errors were made by people who were working in earnest for the good of society.

Given the amount of uncertainty, almost every position was taken on every topic. And on every topic, someone was eventually proved right, and someone else was proved wrong. In some instances, the right people were right for the wrong reasons. In other instances, they had a prescient understanding of the available information.

The people who got it right, for whatever reason, may want to gloat. Those who got it wrong, for whatever reason, may feel defensive and retrench into a position that doesn't accord with the facts. All of this gloating and defensiveness continues to gobble up a lot of social energy and to drive the culture wars, especially on the internet. These discussions are heated, unpleasant and, ultimately, unproductive. In the face of so much uncertainty, getting something right had a hefty element of luck. And, similarly, getting something wrong wasn't a moral failing. Treating pandemic choices as a scorecard on which some people racked up more points than others is preventing us from moving forward.

We have to put these fights aside and declare a pandemic amnesty.

Dr. Oster's kicking over the straw man of "injecting bleach" was itself a particularly egregious example of misinformation, as not a single serious commentator in this debate had ever recommended doing such a thing. But never mind that for now.

Dr. Oster's soothing prose tended to obscure the fact that only one side in this debate had been engaged in censoring and deplatforming its opponents. Only one side had the assistance of psy-ops experts skilled in manipulating people through fear, guilt, and scapegoating. Only one side had the backing of multibillion-dollar drug companies with long records of hiding data and of arrant disregard for the law and arrant disregard for human life. Only one side had the backing of legacy media outlets addicted to drug company advertising in a time of falling ad revenues. Only one side had caused thousands of people to be fired from their jobs for making private medical decisions.

Now, after that side had been spewing out the foulest invective at its opponents, for months and months, Dr. Oster seemed to be saying, in effect, "We all meant well—now let's let bygones be bygones."

The piece touched off a firestorm of criticism on Twitter. YouTube commentator Lauren Chen perhaps said it best:

> Forgiveness usually comes after an apology. I see no apology in this piece. Remember how you encouraged family members to pressure each other and the unvaxxed to be fired? Perhaps a little "I'm sorry for that" would be a good place to start.

A Commitment to Free and Open Debate

On 2 November, the New Civil Liberties Alliance filed suit, demanding AB 2098 be struck down as unconstitutional. The suit (*Høeg v Newsom*) was filed on behalf of Dr. Kheriarty and four other experts. The plaintiffs included California Governor Gavin Newsom and California Attorney General Rob Bronta, as well as the members of the Medical Board of California.

Jenin Younes made this statement:

> California's new 'misinformation' law is the result of an increasingly censorious mentality that has gripped many lawmakers in this country.
>
> That this shocking bill passed through the state legislature and was signed into law by Governor Newsom demonstrates that far too many Americans do not understand the First Amendment. Our country has a strong historical commit-ment to free and open debate and to protect the ability of

those who dissent from the government's view to express their own opinions. We have no doubt that courts will see this unconstitutional law for what it is and strike it down.[387]

The next day, the *Los Angeles Times* ran an article titled "Are the Unvaccinated Still a Danger to the Rest of Us?"[388] After acknowledging that being fully vaccinated confers "just a whiff" of protection against the Omicron variant, the piece served up the same stale old red herring argument, claiming the vax reduces the frequency of severe illness and death due to COVID-19, and called for more boosters—despite the complete lack of long-term data on the safety or effectiveness of repeated booster shots.

Still, the article was quite a comedown for a publication which just months before had called for the "mocking" of the deaths of the unvaccinated.

A Red Trickle?

Mid-term elections were held on Tuesday 8 November. By a narrow margin, Senator Johnson was returned to Washington for a third term.

But the "Red Wave" some had hoped for failed to materialize. The Democrats lost nine seats in the House of Representatives, leaving them a total of 213, while the Republicans gained nine for a total of 222, earning them a solid majority in that chamber. In the Senate, the Republicans lost one seat, leaving them a total of forty-nine, while the Democrats have gained one for a total of forty-nine, along with two more senators from other parties who caucus with the Democrats.

After the election, Senator Krysten Sinema of Arizona announced she was leaving the Democratic Party to become an independent. However, she said she will not be caucusing with the Republicans, and her past record shows that most of the time she has voted with the Democrats. Even if that changes, Vice President Kamala Harris has the power to cast the tie-breaking vote in the Senate, so the Democrats still will have retained control of that body—albeit by the narrowest possible margin.

Missouri v Biden still is pending, as is *Høeg et al. v Newsom*, and *Jackson v Ventavia*. No doubt many more lawsuits will be filed, and no doubt the legal wrangling will drag on for years. The wounds of vaccine injury and vaccine divisiveness (not to mention lockdowns, school closures, and masking of children) will be with us for decades.

Whether the "Pandemic Amnesty" requested by Dr. Oster will be forthcoming remains to be seen.

Some Random Dude on Twitter

Meanwhile, on 14 November , the *Daily Mail* reported that both Pfizer and Moderna have launched trials to determine whether there are any long-term health effects associated with the covid vaccines.[389] The article did not mention that the original trials had been slated to last for two years, and were called off after only a few percent of participants had made it to the six-month mark.

A 19 November article in the *New York Times* noted that the BA.4 and BA.5 variants were already fading into the rear-view mirror, that the new bivalent boosters provided little or no protection against infection for the new BQ.1 and BQ.1.1 variants now circulating, and that the antibodies produced by the new bivalent shots mainly recognize only the original strain of the virus—which is long gone.[390]

Three days later, the *BMJ* ran an article titled "Understanding and Neutralizing Covid-19 Misinformation and Disinformation."[391] An entire treatise on logical fallacies could be written using nothing but examples culled from this piece. Some selections follow:

Flipping the script:

Some [covid skeptic organizations] benefit from generous funding from those opposed to what they term 'big government.'

Arguing from authority:

Inevitably, given the complex technical issues, differentiating fact from fiction can be difficult.

Guilt by association:

This was set in the Brussels Declaration, which was drafted with substantial input from the tobacco companies.

Begging the question:

In times of crisis, people are more susceptible to misinformation, disinformation, and conspiracy theories, probably because their important psychological needs are unfulfilled, leading to frustration.

Straw man argument:

5G technology having deleterious health effects were also mentioned.

More flipping the script:

Given the lack of transparency in allowing academic researchers to examine the potential harms of these platforms

...

In total, the piece mentions the tobacco companies three times but never gets around to telling us that forty-five percent of the candidates and lobbying groups receiving money from Pfizer—the nation's biggest pharmaceutical donor since 2010—have also received money from Altria, the parent company of R.J. Reynolds.[392]

That same day, Anthony Fauci stepped down after fifty-four years of public service, including thirty-eight years as Director of NIAID. At his final press briefing at the White House,[393] he offered these words of advice:

> Are the vaccines safe? That keeps coming up. Overwhelmingly, it should be off the table. There have been 13 billion doses of a COVID-19 vaccine that have been distributed worldwide, hundreds of millions in the United States. And there's robust safety monitoring systems that are in place. And clearly, an extensive body of information indicates that they're safe.
>
> Next: Are they effective? And I believe you are all aware of this. If you look at the striking data, overwhelmingly show the effectiveness of vaccines, particularly in preventing severe illness and deaths.
>
> So my final message and my final message—may be the final message I give you from this podium—is that: Please, for your own safety, for that of your family, get your updated COVID-19 shot as soon as you're eligible to protect yourself, your family, and your community.

Ashish Jha, White House Coronavirus Response Coordinator, was also present, and he had this to say:

> For a majority of Americans, this is going to be a once-a-year shot. One covid shot, just like the flu shot.
>
> Please, don't wait. Get your covid shot. Get your flu shot. That's why God gave you two arms. You can get one in each arm if you want.

White House Press Secretary Karine Jean-Pierre summed up matters thusly:

> So I started my comment by reminding everybody that America's physicians, like the real leaders of American medicine—the people you trust for your cancer care and your heart care and your pediatrics care—are out there telling you you need to go get a vaccine. You can decide to trust America's physicians, or you can trust some random dude on Twitter. Those are your choices.

The very next day, Dr. Fauci was deposed as part of the *Missouri v Biden* lawsuit. That evening, Attorney Jenin Younes tweeted:

> One of my favorite quotes from Fauci's deposition today: "I have a very busy day job running a six billion dollar institute. I don't have time to worry about things like the Great Barrington Declaration."

When I learned Dr. Fauci was being deposed, all I could think was *It's about bloody time.*

CHAPTER SIXTEEN

Alleged Crimes and Wrongdoing

December 2022 - January 2023

We're Going to Look

Missouri v Biden may not be the only problem Dr. Fauci is facing. On Tuesday 13 December, Florida Governor Ron DeSantis (who had just won his bid for re-election by a wide margin) announced that he was forming a state committee to evaluate policy recommendations from federal health agencies. That same day he announced he was requesting a statewide grand jury to investigate alleged crimes and wrongdoing related to the covid vaccines. [394]

Florida State Surgeon General Joseph Ladapo announced he would work with doctors at the University of Florida to study cases of sudden death following administration of the vax, telling reporters:

> It's a question that I'm sure keeps the CEO's of Pfizer and Moderna up late at night hoping no one ever looks. We're going to look here in Florida.

The *Washington Post* decried these moves, averring that "there's no evidence that the vaccines have led to widespread medical issues, much less death."[395] As proof, they pointed to a study which used county-level party affiliation as a proxy for behaviors believed to decrease transmission of the virus—masking and social distancing as well as vaxxing—and which found that Republican-leaning counties in Ohio and Florida had higher rates of COVID-19 mortality than Democrat-leaning ones after the vax was rolled out.[396] The *WaPo* article did not mention that the absolute increase in excess deaths was tiny—less than one in a thousand—and the study authors themselves attributed just ten percent of this to vaccination status.

Furthermore, the study did not even look at the only statistic which matters in the end—all-cause mortality. Are fewer people dying of the covid in Democrat-leaning counties because they are dying of the vax? There is no way of knowing from reading the paper.

Four days later, the *WaPo* reaffirmed its position,[397] citing this statement:

> Over the course of this deadly pandemic, mRNA vaccines have saved hundreds of thousands of lives, tens of billions of dollars in health care costs, and enabled people worldwide to go about their lives more freely.

That statement was issued by Pfizer.

Disturbing Findings

On 19 December, a study by the Cleveland Clinic[398] showed that efficacy of the bivalent booster was just thirty percent, far below the minimum value of fifty percent promised by then-FDA-commissioner Stephen Hahn, way back in August of 2020. How long even this puny effect can be expected to last is an open question, given that maximum follow-up time was ninety-eight days.

Even more disturbingly, the likelihood of infection after the booster shot *increased* with the number of previous injections. Those who received the booster shot after three or more prior doses had three times the likelihood of subsequent infection than those who had none. In other words, there was a dose-dependent relationship between the number of prior shots and the likelihood of infection. This sort of thing usually is considered proof of a cause-and-effect relationship.

In fairness, there may have been some potential confounders here. Perhaps those got the most prior shots were the ones most at risk for COVID-19. But the researchers themselves nixed that idea, noting that almost all the subjects (Cleveland Clinic employees all) were young and healthy, all were eligible to receive three or more prior shots, and all had every opportunity to do so.

That same day, a team of Japanese researchers provided a possible explanation for all this.[399] Their paper described the latest variant of the coronavirus, called XBB, which came into being via genetic recombination of two other strains. The new strain was more infective than prior strains, and also much more resistant to antibodies produced in response to the bivalent booster shot.

As always, the wisdom of trying to vaccinate our way out of a pandemic was not questioned.

Official Causes of Death

Also that same day, Senator Johnson dispatched yet another oversight letter, this one to Lieutenant General Ronald J. Place, Director of the Defense Health Agency. As usual, the senator did not mince words:

> Despite the unprecedented number of adverse events and deaths associated with the COVID-19 vaccines on the Vaccine Adverse Event Reporting System, this administra-

tion has failed to provide full and transparent information on vaccine safety to Congress and to the public.

Although the Biden Administration's COVID-19 vaccine mandate for the military will end with the signing of the Fiscal Year 2023 National Defense Authorization Act, my efforts to uncover and expose the vaccines' harmful effects on our service members will continue. The brave men and women who serve our country deserve to know the truth about the short and long-term health effects these mandated vaccines will have on the rest of their lives.

Senator Johnson requested the agency provide data by year from 2017 onward for the number of claims filed related to these diagnoses:

- Breast cancer
- Demyelinating
- Female infertility
- Guillain-Barré syndrome
- Hypertension
- Malignant neoplasms of the esophagus, digestive organs, and the thyroid and other endocrine glands
- Migraines
- Multiple sclerosis
- Myocarditis
- Pericarditis
- Pulmonary embolism
- Ovarian dysfunction
- Tachycardia
- Testicular cancer

The senator also requested that the agency provide the number of service members who had at least one dose of the vax, and for those members a monthly breakdown of the number of claims for each of the above-mentioned diagnoses filed between January 2020 to the present. Finally, he asked for the number of service members who died within seven days after receiving the shot, along with any preexisting medical conditions and the official cause of death.

Senator Johnson requested that the agency reply to his concerns no later than 9 January 2023.

This Tweet Cannot be Shared, Replied to, or Liked

Meanwhile, efforts continued to uncover the breadth and depth of government censorship campaigns against anyone questioning the official narrative. The previous October, Tesla CEO and billionaire Elon Musk acquired Twitter and offered to make that company's secret files available to any researcher who wanted to look at them—provided they made their findings public on Twitter first. Author David Zweig availed himself of the opportunity, and his account, published the day after Christmas, told a tale of Twitter users—some of them eminently credentialed experts— having their contributions suppressed for communicating opinions and/or truthful information.

On 21 March 2021 Harvard epidemiologist Martin Kulldorff (who, as you should recall, was one of the authors of the Great Barrington Declaration) had tweeted the following:

> Thinking that everyone should be vaccinated is as scientifically flawed as thinking nobody should. covid vaccines are important for older, high-risk people, and their care-takers. Those with prior natural infection do not need it. Nor children.

Dr. Kulldorff's tweet was the opinion of an internationally recognized expert, and one that was in line with official guidelines in numerous other countries. Nevertheless, Twitter slapped the tweet with a "false information" label which prevented users from liking, replying, or sharing, in turn diminishing the ability of other users to see and share the tweet—undercutting the very reason to be on the platform.

Another user, who styles herself Kelly K, had a Tweet similarly restricted for sharing official CDC data demonstrating that COVID-19 is not a leading cause of death among children. Jay Bhattacharya, who like Dr. Kulldorff was one of the authors of the Great Barrington Declaration, was placed on a blacklist secretly, ensuring his posts would be positioned lower in the feed of other users as well as denying him the ability respond to or even see the accusations against him. And Andrew Bostom, a physician from Rhode Island, was kicked off the platform after sharing a peer-reviewed paper demonstrating that the Pfizer shot lowered sperm count in men.

Breakthrough

On the third day of the New year, the *Epoch Times* reported that the CDC had finally gotten around to releasing the results of the Proportional Report Ratio analysis they had promised back in January of 2021.[400] The results, as mentioned earlier, were eye-opening.

The analysis covered adverse events reported from 14 December 2020 through 29 July 2022. Remember the PRR for a given event has to be at least 2:1 to be considered a "signal." There were over seven hundred such signals. Here is just a partial list:

- Pulmonary: Lung opacity, increased respiratory rate, pulmonary pain, acute respiratory failure, decreased oxygen saturation, atypical pneumonia

- Neurological: Ischemic stroke, cerebellar stroke, anosmia, ageusia, Bell's palsy, electric shock sensation

- Cardiovascular: myocarditis, pericarditis, thrombectomy, increased blood pressure, pulmonary thrombosis, left ventricular failure, acute cardiac failure, stent placement, acute left ventricular failure, intracardiac thrombus, right ventricular dilation, portal vein thrombosis, implantable cardiac monitor insertion, myocardial strain, mesenteric vein thrombosis, jugular vein thrombosis, thromboembolectomy, coronary angioplasty, vascular dementia, embolic stroke, hypertensive emergency, coronary artery thrombosis, pulmonary infarction, increased troponin level, acute myocardial infarction, coronary artery stent insertion, deep vein thrombosis, coronary artery occlusion, cardiorespiratory arrest

- Hepatic: Liver injury, elevated liver enzymes, liver disorder, hepatic mass, hepatic cirrhosis

- Renal: End-stage renal disease, chronic kidney disease, acute kidney injury

In Chapter Two we discussed the possible link between the spike protein and cancer. The CDC analysis found signals for colon cancer, metastatic breast cancer, thyroid cancer, lung adenocarcinoma, pancreatic carcinoma, metastases to lymph nodes, metastases to central nervous system, metastases to liver, and metastases to bone.

We also discussed the possible link between the spike protein and heightened immune response. The CDC analysis found signals for paranasal sinus inflammation, gastrointestinal inflammation, breast inflammation, inner ear inflammation, colitis, epididymitis, peritonitis, pancreatitis, glossitis, mastitis, cutaneous vasculitis, endocarditis, hand dermatitis, appendicitis, giant cell arteritis, diverticulitis, pneumonitis, and autoimmune hepatitis.

In Chapters Thirteen and Fourteen we discussed possible reproductive effects of the vax. The CDC analysis linked the mRNA shots to heavy menstrual bleeding, intermenstrual bleeding, polymenorrhea, post-menopausal hemorrhage, abnormal uterine bleeding, oligomenorrhea, menstrual disorder, irregular menstruation, premenstrual pain, premenstrual syndrome, ovulation disorder, hypomenorrhea, and amenorrhea.

Miscellaneous effects included decreased body height, superinfection, critical illness, amyloidosis, hospitalization, and multiple organ dysfunction syndrome. Not to mention death.

But bigger than the signal for any of these was the one for "serious vaccine breakthrough infection," for which the PRR was a whopping 315 times that of comparator products. So much for the vaunted "efficacy" of these nostrums.

In an accompanying letter, the CDC told the *Times* that the results "generally corroborated the findings from Empirical Bayesian Data Mining, revealing no additional unexpected safety signals." That is not terribly reassuring.

No Scientific Justification

Six days later, former *New York Times* reporter Alex Berenson reported on his Substack[401] that former FDA Commissioner and current Pfizer board member Scott Gottlieb had demanded that Twitter take action against Brett Giror, a bioweapons expert and *former Acting FDA Commissioner*, who correctly pointed out on that platform that natural immunity to covid is superior to vaccine-enforced immunity. On 27 August 2021, Dr. Giror tweeted this message:

> It's now clear that #COVID19 natural immunity is superior to #vaccine immunity, by A LOT. There's no scientific justification for #vax proof if a person had prior infection. @CDCDirector@POTUS must follow the science. If no previous infection? Get vaccinated!

Dr. Gottlieb, who is paid $365,000 per year for his services to Pfizer, took exception to Dr. Giror's disparagement of Pfizer's products. He complained to a Twitter lobbyist, who forwarded the complaint to Twitter's "Strategic Response Team," which determined that the tweet had not violated company policy. Nonetheless, Twitter flagged the post as "misleading," preventing almost anyone from seeing it.

Rethinking Next-Generation Vaccines

Four days after that, a review paper authored by no less a luminary than Anthony Fauci (along with two of his colleagues) appeared in the journal *Cell Host & Microbe*.[402] Titled "Rethinking Next-Generation Vaccines," the piece began by pointing out challenges in developing effective vaccines for COVID-19 or influenza, as opposed to long-established vaccines for such illnesses as measles, mumps, or rubella. The authors noted that while the viruses that cause all of these diseases enter the body via the upper respiratory tract, the viruses that cause measles, mumps, and rubella have a long incubation time, during which they enter multiple body compartments including the circulatory system, giving the body time to develop effective humoral immunity (immunity conferred by antibodies in the blood). By contrast, the coronavirus and the influenza virus multiply rapidly and reach peak infectivity before the body even has time to mount an effective humoral immune response. Moreover, the genomes for the viruses that cause measles, mumps, and rubella have overlapping reading frames, enabling the same sequence of RNA to be read in multiple ways and therefore code for multiple proteins. This makes these viruses relatively resistant to mutations. The coronavirus and the influenza virus are under no such constraint, and so more readily evolve mutations, including ones that enable them to escape the body's acquired immunity.

In plain English: Dr. Fauci and his co-authors were telling us that the experts knew going in that it was highly unlikely any vaccine for the coronavirus would stop transmission—the linchpin of the justification for inveigling or coercing hundreds of millions to get these shots.

They knew.

The Summing Up

1) The evidence purporting to demonstrate the mRNA "vaccines" are safe and effective was manufactured by three companies, one of which has a long history of hiding data and of an arrant disregard for the law and arrant disregard for human life, and the other two which had no products at all on the market before 2020 and now have a single product apiece, with billions and billions of dollars riding on that product.

2) The studies that served as the basis for emergency use authorization of these products showed no reduction in deaths and an increase in serious adverse events. The studies also did not measure transmission of the virus, and they were not powered to demonstrate benefits in vulnerable populations such as pregnant women or immunocompromised or elderly patients.

3) The primary endpoint for these studies—covid infection of any severity—cannot be believed since the investigators did not count cases of covid arising within four weeks after the administration of the first dose (or six weeks, in the case of the Moderna product)—and we have seen evidence that these products increase the rate of covid infection in at least the first few days after administration.

4) These studies were supposed to involve tens of thousands of participants and go on for two years, and were cut off

after only a small percentage of participants made it to the six-month mark. Thus, these products were approved without any RCT data pertaining to the long-term benefits or harms.

5) Hundreds of millions of people were induced or coerced into taking these products without being advised of any of this.

6) FDA originally intended to take seventy-five years to release the full Pfizer trial data, and relented only because of a court order. The full Moderna trial data still has not been released.

7) Since these products came on to the market, reports to VAERS of serious adverse events (including death) believed to be associated with the spike protein have skyrocketed.

8) CDC promised to carry out signal detection analysis of VAERS data beginning in January of 2021. When they finally released the results in January of 2023 (after months and months of dissembling), the analysis showed safety signals for hundreds of different categories of adverse events, including death.

9) FDA promised to carry out signal detection analysis of VAERS data, and either they did not do so or they have not released the results.

10) Since these products came on to the market, reports to DMED of serious adverse events known to be associated with the spike protein have skyrocketed.

11) DMED data for the years 2016-2019 appear to have undergone manipulations of an unspecified nature, with the effect of diminishing the relative size of the 2021 increase in adverse events known to be associated with the spike protein. No satisfactory explanation has been forthcoming.

12) Official guidelines and regulations contain multiple sources of bias toward overcounting cases, hospitalizations, and deaths due to COVID-19.

13) The efficacy of the mRNA shots in preventing covid infection fades quickly, with one recent study reporting negative efficacy five months after the booster shot.

14) The waning efficacy of these products have prompted the FDA to recommend repeated booster shots, despite the complete lack of any long-term data on the effects of repeated inundations of the body with the toxic spike protein.

15) A variety government agencies have engaged in active attempts to shut down dissenting views on the handling of the pandemic on social media.

* * *

As for myself: after my stroke I told people I felt good as new, and for a while this was true, but that is no longer the case. The dizzy spells have become more and more frequent, and I now am dealing with memory lapses I did not have before I got the booster shot.

Still, as I said, compared to a lot of people I got off lightly.

Neither Moderna nor VAERS have followed up on my adverse event reports.

As one of Academia's caste of perma-temps, I no longer teach at either of the two institutions that required me to get the shot as a condition of my continued employment.

* * *

I asked Dr. Healy, What are the lessons to be learned from all this? Here is what he had to say:

> At this stage, I don't know that anyone's in a good position to know what the lessons are. I mean, there's a bunch of things that happened. First of all, you've got gene therapies been passed off as vaccines. We need to know exactly why that happened. We've got scientists, supposedly—people portraying themselves as scientists—saying that the immunity you get from these new products is better than natural immunity. Now this is just unbelievable. This is just not so. I mean, this is just crazy.
>
> So why were "respectable" people saying these things and why was the rest of the field—a lot of people who should have been speaking up and saying, Well, look, that's just plain wrong—why were all these people who ought to have been speaking up, not speaking up?

Epilogue

It was the day after Thanksgiving, an unseasonably warm afternoon, the rolling hills and dales of Washington County forming a viridescent backdrop to the last remaining golden leaves of autumn still clinging to the trees. Two years had elapsed since I had gone for that hastily interrupted stroll with my nephew and nieces and now I had come full circle, literally. They're two years older now, and it took some coaxing to induce them to accompany their uncle on his peregrinations.

My wife and I had driven up the night before, and the kids' mom had served up a delicious feast, and over dinner I lectured them on randomized controlled trials and the placebo effect, and also on the discovery of insulin, and the youngest child, a girl, piped up "Uncle Patrick, you're like a living Wikipedia."

Now we were out and about, strolling down the smooth blacktop lanes past acres of manicured lawns when we spotted a couple, a man and a woman, standing in their driveway. They smiled and waved and greeted us, and we returned their greetings. No fearful avoidance of one another, no muzzles converting the human visage into a cold insectoid gaze—just human beings, sampling the joys of being human. It occurred to me that as a people we seem to be developing antibodies to the climate of fear we have been saturated with for the past almost three years. That was a comforting thought.

We reached the end of a cul-de-sac and stood there for a while, gazing at the blue hills in the distance. A cool breeze blew through, presaging the frigid temperatures forecast for that evening. The middle child, a girl, complained of feeling cold, and so I removed my jacket and draped it over her shoulders.

"Say thank you," her younger sister admonished her, and she did so.

It was time to start heading back. As we made our way back to the house, I reflected on the long sweep of history.

Since time immemorial, nations vanquished other nations and built empires. And the ones that weren't good at it got stomped on by the ones that were. You either grew or you died. This was a moral imperative.

It would seem that this process has been completed. The world has been conquered. Little kids living in mud huts in African villages are now online (I have seen this). There are no more spots on the map marked "Here Be Tygers." The only terrain left for would-be tyrants to subjugate is our own bodies. And in an era in which most of our physical labor (and increasing amounts of our mental labor) are performed by machines, many of us have less value to our rulers as soldiers or workers than we do as consumers of medical interventions.

Power no longer comes from land tenure. It doesn't even come from owning a factory. It comes from manipulating the language of science, and the appearance of science, in order to control people.

Our overlords no longer talk in terms of breeding master races, or building empires upon which the sun never sets. Instead they speak in much more dulcet tones. This is a very good sign—it means they are afraid of us. And nowhere is that fear displayed more rawly than in the pathetic mewling of the legacy media that "You must not do your own research when it comes to science"—the Twenty-First Century equivalent of "Pay no attention to the man behind the curtain."

This is a golden moment. We have the opportunity to seize power from our rulers and use it to make over society not from the top down but from the bottom up—building institutions and communities that operate on a human scale and do a better job of meeting actual human needs. That is the kind of Great Reset we could all get behind. I don't claim to know all the details of what that would look like, but I am happy to have that conversation with anyone who wants to have it.

Flatulent babbling about "Hacking the software of life" needs to be replaced with a sense of awe and wonder at the complexity of the human organism—the product of over five hundred million years of evolution—along with an intelligent awareness that our lives have meaning only within the context of a larger human society, and an acceptance of our mortality.

Vaccines were not even on my radar before the covid pandemic began. That is no longer the case. I now have questions I did not have before—and that is all I am going to say about the matter today.

Of course, these mRNA shots should not even be called "vaccines" at all—but never mind that for now. To whatever extent people are turning away from truly life-saving vaccines, the drugmakers, public health officials, and their apologists and shills in the legacy media and the entertainment industry have only themselves to blame. Arguments from authority, coercion, threats, censorship, deplatforming, fearmongering, vulgar abuse, free donuts, or (perhaps worst of all) fake "empathy" and condescending attempts to assuage our fears are just not going to cut it. There is an urgent need for the "experts" to engage with the rest of us as responsible citizens, with facts and data, and to admit to their past transgressions.

But that is not going to happen unless we make it happen.

The four of us ascended the driveway in front of their home, eagerly awaiting what lay in store for us—hot chocolate around the kitchen table, and the shelter of each other.

References

ABC News. "Girlfriend Believes Chantix Contributed to Texas Musician's Death." September 19, 2007. https://abcnews.go.com/GMA/OnCall/story?id=3623085&page=1

Adams, Ben. "A Tale of 2 (Bio) Cities: Moderna Tops $100B Valuation, Matching GlaxoSmithKline." *Fierce Biotech*, July 15, 2021. https://www.fiercebiotech.com/biotech/a-tale-two-bio-cities-moderna-tops-100b-valuation-matching-glaxosmithkline

Al-Aly, Ziyad, Benjamin Bowe, and Yan Xie. "Long Covid after Breakthrough SARS-CoV-2 Infection." *Nature Medicine* 28, no. 7 (July 2022): 1461-1467. https://doi.org/10.1038/s41591-022-01840-0

Alexanderson, Kristina, Rochelle Ann Burgess, Laura Bear, Reinhard Busse, David Fishman, Lynn R. Goldman, Adam Hamdy, et al. "John Snow Memorandum." October 14, 2020. https://www.johnsnowmemo.com/john-snow-memo.html

Altarawneh, Heba, Hiam Chemaitelly, Patrick Tang, Mohammed R. Hasan, Suelen Qassim, Houssein H. Ayoub, Sawsan AlMukdad, et al. "Protection by Prior Infection against SARS-CoV-2 Reinfection with the Omicron Variant." medRxiv preprint, January 6, 2022. https://www.medrxiv.org/content/10.1101/2022.01.05.22268782v1

Alter, Ethan. "Arnold Schwarzenegger's 'Screw Your Freedom' Remark Leads to a Sponsorship Loss." Yahoo Entertainment, August 24, 2021. https://www.yahoo.com/entertainment/arnold-schwarzenegger-sponsorship-loss-184606881.html

Alvergne, Alexandra, Gabriella Kountourides, M. Austin Argentieri, Lisa Agyen, Natalie Rogers, Gemma C. Sharp, Jacqueline A. Maybin, and Zusanna Olszewska. "Characterizing Menstrual Cycle Changes Occurring after SARS-CoV-2 Vaccination." medRxiv preprint, October 12, 2021. https:// www.medrxiv.org/content/10.1101/2021.10.11.21264863v1

Anonymous. "I Am Struggling to Understand Why Patients Decide Not to Get the Covid Vaccine." *BMJ* 2021;375:n3152

Arnsdorf, Isaac. "DeSantis Reverses Himself on Coronavirus Vaccines, Moves to Right of Trump." *Washington Post,* December 17, 2022.

Arvin, Ann M., Katja Fink, Michael A. Schmid, Andrea Cathcart, Roberto Spreafico, Colin Havenar-Daughton, Antonio Lanzavecchia, Davide Corti, and Herbert W. Virgin. "A Perspective on Potential Antibody-Dependent Enhancement of SARS-CoV-2." *Nature* 584, no. 7821 (August 20, 2020): 353-363. https://doi.org/10.1038/s41586-020-2538-8

Associated Press. "FDA Investigates Quit-Smoking Drug." *New York Times,* November 21, 2007.

Associated Press. "Chantix, Smoking Cessation Drug, Blamed in Murder-Suicide." *Oregonian,* December 1, 2013. https://www.oregonlive.com/pacific-northwest-news/2013/11/chantix_smoking_cessation_drug.html

Associated Press. "NYC Fires More Than 1,000 Workers Over Vaccine Mandate." *New York Times,* February 14, 2022.

Axios. "Pfizer CEO Says He Would Have Released Vaccine Data before Election if Possible." November 9, 2020. https://www.axios.com/2020/11/09/pfizer-ceo-says-he-wouldve-released-vaccine-data-before-election-if-possible

BBC. "Covid Vaccine: How Many People Are Vaccinated in the UK?" March 4, 2022. https://www.bbc.com/news/health-55274833

Bardosh, Kevin, Allison Krug, Euzebiusz Jamrozik, Trudo Lemmons, Candjur Licjur, Salmaan Keshavjee, Vinay Prasad, Martin Makary, Stefan Baral, and Tracy Beth Høeg. "Covid-19 Vaccine Boosters for Young Adults: A Risk-Benefit Assessment and Five Ethical Arguments against Vaccine Mandates at Universities." SSRN, September 12, 2022. https://papers.ssrn.com/sol3/papers.cfm?abstract_id=4206070

Baxby, Derrick. "Edward Jenner's Inquiry after 200 Years." *BMJ* 318, no. 7180 (February 6, 1999): 390. https://doi.org/10.1136/bmj.318.7180.390

Beaumont, Oliver, David Doukhan, Pauline Théveniaud, Henri Vernet, and Marcelo Wesfried. "Europe, Vaccination, Présidentielle … Emmanuel Macron Se Livre à nos Lecteurs." *Le Parisien*, January 4, 2022. https://www.leparisien.fr/politique/europe-vaccination-presidentielle-emmanuel-macron-se-livre-a-nos-lecteurs-04-01-2022-2KVQ3ESNSREABMTD-WR25OMGWEA.php?ts=1641326582881

Bella, Timothy. "Jimmy Kimmel Suggests Hospitals Shouldn't Treat Unvaccinated People." *Washington Post,* September 8, 2021.

Berenson, Alex. "Pfizer Loses One Remedy for Its Slump." *New York Times*, April 7, 2005, C1.

Berenson, Alex. *Pandemia: How Coronavirus Hysteria Took over Our Government, Rights, and Lives.* Washington DC: Regnery Publishing, November 30, 2021.

Berenson, Alex. "From the Twitter Files: Pfizer Board Member Scott Gottlieb Secretly Pressed Twitter to Hide Posts Challenging His Company's Massively Profitable Covid Jabs." Substack, January 9, 2023. https://alexberenson.substack.com/p/pfizer-board-member-scott-gottlieb

Bernal, Jamie Lopez, Nick Andrews, Charlotte Gower, Julia Stowe, Chris Robertson, Elise Tessier, Ruth Simmons, et al. "Early Effectiveness of COVID-19 Vaccination with BNT162b mRNA Vaccine and ChAdOx1 Adenovirus Vector Vaccine on Symptomatic Disease, Hospitalizations, and Mortality in Older Adults in England." medRxiv preprint, March 2, 2021. https://www.medrxiv.org/content/10.1101/2021.03.01.21252652v1

Bhopal, Sunil S., Jayshree Bagaria, Bayanne Olabi, and Raj Bhopal. "Children and Young People Remain at Low Risk of COVID-19 Mortality." *Lancet: Child and Adolescent Health* 5, March 10, 2021. https://doi.org/10.1016/S2352-4642(21)00066-3

Bill and Melinda Gates Foundation. "Committed Grants: CNN.com." September 2020. https://www.gatesfoundation.org/about/committed-grants/2020/09/inv004478

BioNTech. "BioNTech Signs Collaborative Agreement with Pfizer to Develop mRNA-Based Vaccines for Prevention of Influenza." August 16, 2018. https://biontechse.gcs-web.com/news-releases/news-release-details/biontech-signs-collaboration-agreement-pfizer-develop-mrna-based

BioNTech. "Biopharma Leaders Unite to Stand with Science." September 8, 2020. https://www.globenewswire.com/news-release/2020/09/08/2089875/0/en/Biopharma-Leaders-Unite-to-Stand-with-Science.html

BioNTech. "BioNTech Announces Fourth Quarter and Full Year 2021 Financial Results and Corporate Update." March 30, 2022. https://investors.biontech.de/news-releases/news-release-details/biontech-announces-fourth-quarter-and-full-year-2021-financial

BioNTech. "Pipeline." Accessed May 28, 2022. https://www.biontech.com/content/dam/corporate/pdf/20220330_BiontechPipeline.pdf

Block, Jennifer. "Vaccinating People Who Have Had Covid-19: Why Doesn't Natural Immunity Count?" *BMJ* 2021;374n:n2101

Blow, Charles M. "I'm Furious at the Unvaccinated." *New York Times*, December 8, 2021.

Boucau, Julie, Caitlin Marino, James Regan, Rockib Uddin, Manish C. Choudhary, Geoffrey Chen, Ashley M. Strudwisch, et al. "Duration of Shedding of Culturable Virus in SARS-CoV-2 Omicron (BA.1) Infection." *New England Journal of Medicine* 387, no. 3 (July 21, 2022): 275-277. https://www.nejm.org/doi/full/10.1056/nejmc2202092

Bourla, Albert. *Moonshot.* New York: Harper Collins, March 8, 2022.

Breggin, Peter Roger, and Ginger Ross Breggin. *COVID-19 and the Global Predators: We Are the Prey.* Ithaca: Lake Edge Press, September 30, 2021.

Brooks, Megan. "Keep Chantix Black Box Warning, FDA Panel Says." Medscape, October 17, 2014. https://www.medscape.com/viewarticle/833402

Brown, Catherine M., Johanna Vostok, Hilary Johnson, Megan Burns, Radhika Ghapure, Samira Sami, Rebecca T. Sabo, et al. "Outbreak of SARS-CoV-2 Infections, Including COVID-19 Vaccine Breakthrough Infections, Associated with Large Public Gatherings—Barnstable County, Massachusetts, July 2021." *Morbidity and Mortality Weekly Report* 70, (July 30, 2021). https://www.cdc.gov/mmwr/volumes/70/wr/mm7031e2.htm

Brown, Eric L., and Heather T. Essigmann. "Original Antigenic Sin: The Downside of Immunological Memory and Implications for COVID-19." *mSphere* 6, no. 2 (March 10, 2021): 1-6. https://doi.org/10/1128/mSphere.00056-21

Bruno, Roxana, Peter A. McCullough, Teresa Forcades i Vila, Alexandra Henrion Caude, Teresa García-Gasca, Galina P. Zaitzeva, Sally Priester, et al. "SARS-CoV-2 Mass Vaccination: Urgent Questions on Vaccine Safety That Demand Answers from International Health Agencies, Regulatory Authorities, Governments, and Vaccine Developers." May 18, 2021.

Bump, Philip. "DeSantis Again Threatens Legal Action with an Eye on 2024." *Washington Post*, December 13, 2022.

Burdick, Suzanne. "'God Gave Us Two Arms—One for the Flu Shot, One for the Covid Shot.'" *Defender*, September 7, 2022. https://childrenshealthdefense.org/defender/ashish-jha-flu-shot-covid-shot-white-house-covid-response/

CBS News. "2nd Quit-Smoking Drug Gets FDA's OK." May 11, 2006. https://www.cbsnews.com/news/2nd-quit-smoking-drug-gets-fdas-ok/

CBS News. "New York City Mayor Bill DeBlasio Promotes a New Incentive to Get Vaccinated: Shake Shack." May 13, 2021. https://www.cbsnews.com/video/new-york-city-mayor-bill-de-blasio-covid-19-vaccine-free-shake-shack/#x

CBS New York. "Mayor Adams Says Professional Athletes, Performers Now Exempt from Vaccine Mandate." March 24, 2022. https://www.cbsnews.com/newyork/live-updates/eric-adams-vaccine-mandate-pro-athletes-performers-kyrie-irving/

CDC. "Meeting of the Advisory Committee on Immunization Practices (ACIP)." May 12, 2021.

CDC. "COVID-19 VaSt Work Group Report." May 17, 2021. https://www.cdc.gov/vaccines/acip/work-groups-vast/report-2021-05-17.html?CDC_

AA_refVal=https%3A%2F%2Fwww.cdc.gov%2Fvaccines%2Facip%2F-work-groups-vast%2Ftechnical-report-2021-05-17.html

CDC. "SARS-CoV-2 B.1.1.529 (Omicron) Variant—United States, December 1-8, 2021." *Morbidity and Mortality Weekly Report* 70, no. 50 (December 17, 2021): 1731-1734. December 17, 2021. https://www.cdc.gov/mmwr/volumes/70/wr/mm7050e1.htm

CDC. "Weekly Updates by Select Demographic and Geographic Characteristics: Provisional Death Counts for Coronavirus Disease 2019 (COVID-19): Comorbidities and Other Conditions." June 2, 2022. https://www.cdc.gov/nchs/nvss/vsrr/covid_weekly/index.htm#Comorbidities

CDC. "Frequently Asked Questions about COVID-19 Vaccination." Updated July 11, 2022. https://www.cdc.gov/coronavirus/2019-ncov/vaccines/faq.html

CDC. "Long Covid or Post-COVID Conditions." Updated September 1, 2022. https://www.cdc.gov/coronavirus/2019ncov/long-term-effects/index.html

CDC. "Rates of COVID-19 Cases or Deaths by Age Groups and Vaccination Status and Second Booster Dose." Updated October 21, 2022. https://data.cdc.gov/Public-Health-Surveillance/Rates-of-COVID-19-Cases-or-Deaths-by-Age-Group-and/d6p8-wqjm

Callard, Felicity, and Elise Perego. "How and Why Patients Made Long Covid." *Social Science and Medicine* 268, (January 2021). https://doi.org/10.1016/j.socscimed2020.113426

Canas, Liane, Erika Molteni, Jie Deng, Carole H. Sudre, Benjamin Murray, Eric Kerfoot, Michela Antonelli, et al. "Profiling Post-Covid Syndrome across Different Variants of SARS-CoV-2." medRxiv preprint, July 31, 2022. https://www.medrxiv.org/content/10.1101/2022.07.28.22278159v1

Cedars Sinai. "New Data Show COVID-19 Vaccine Does Not Raise Stroke Risk." August 24, 2022. https://www.cedars-sinai.org/newsroom/new-data-shows-covid-19-vaccine-does-not-raise-stroke-risk/

Cheng, Derek. "Coronavirus: Jacinda Ardern Dismisses Nationwide Lockdown Speculation on Social Media." *New Zealand Herald*, March 18, 2020. https://www.nzherald.co.nz/nz/coronavirus-jacinda-ardern-dismisses-nationwide-lockdown-speculation-on-social-media/I2FTKPSA36LJIDNLB-FIYECXDHM

Chung, Frank. "Pfizer Did Not Know Whether Covid Vaccine Stopped Transmission before Rollout, Executive Admits." news.com, October 13, 2022. https://www.news.com.au/technology/science/human-body/pfizer-did-not-know-whether-covid-vaccine-stopped-transmission-before-rollout-executive-admits/news-story/f307f28f794e173ac017a62784fec414

Cincinnati Children's. "Myocarditis in Children." Updated April 2019. https://www.cincinnatichildrens.org/health/m/myocarditis

Coalition for Epidemic Preparedness Innovations. "CEPI to Fund Three Programmes to Develop Three Vaccines against the Novel Coronavirus, nCoV-2019." January 23, 2020. https://cepi.net/news_cepi/cepi_to_fund_three_programmes_to_develop_three_vaccines_against_the_novel Coronavirus, nCoV-2019/

Coronavirus Study Group. "Severe Acute Respiratory Syndrome-Related Coronavirus: The Species and Its Viruses." February 11, 2020. https://www.biorxiv.org/content/10.1101/2020.02.07.937862v1

Crawford, Mathew. "Defining Away Vaccine Safety Signals 5: The DMED Data 'Glitch' Revealed?" Substack, March 22, 2022. https://roundingtheearth.substack.com/p/defining-away-vaccine-safety-signals-82f

Crawford, Mathew. "Defining Away Vaccine Safety Signals 7: Fact Checkers Miss the Point." Substack, April 3, 2022. https://roundingtheearth.substack.com/p/defining-away-vaccine-safety-signals-a10

Cyranoski, David. "Why Emergency Covid-Vaccine Approvals Pose a Dilemma for Scientists." *Nature*, November 23, 2020. https://www.nature.com/articles/d41586-020-03219-y

Czeisler, Mark E., Rashin I. Lane, Emiko Petrosky, Joshua F. Wiley, Aleta Christensen, Rashid Njai, Matthew D. Weaver, et al. "Mental Health, Substance Abuse, and Suicidal Ideation during the COVID-19 Pandemic—United States, June 24-30, 2020." *Morbidity and Mortality Weekly Report* 69, no. 32 (August 14, 2020): 1049-1057. https://www.cdc.gov/mmwr/volumes/69/wr/mm6932a1.htm

Czopek, Madison. "No, COVID-19 Vaccines Aren't Responsible for an Increase in Deaths." PolitiFact, February 11, 2022. https://www.politifact.com/factchecks/2022/feb/11/blog-posting/no-covid-19-vaccines-arent-responsible-increase-de/

Daily Mail. "Father Who Murdered His Family Had Been on Anti-Smoking Medication That Caused Depression." April 6, 2011. https://www.dailymail.co.uk/news/article-1373983/Father-murdered-family-quitting-smoking-medication-caused-depression.html

Davis, Hannah E., Gina S. Assaf, Lisa McCorkell, Hannah Wei, Ryan J. Low, Yochai Re'em, Signe Redfield, Jared P. Austin, and Athena Akrami. "Characterizing Long Covid in an International Cohort: 7 Months of Symptoms and Their Impact." *EClinical Medicine* 38, (2021). https://doi.org/10.1016/eclinm.2021.101019

Day, Michael. "Covid-19: Stronger Warnings Are Needed to Curb Socializing after Vaccination, Say Doctors and Behavioural Scientists." *BMJ* 2021;372:n783

Devlin, Hannah, and Richard Adams. "Covid Resurgent across UK with Infections in over-70s at All-Time High." *Guardian*, March 18, 2022.

Dickler, Jessica. "Krispy Kreme Doubles Its Free Donut Incentive for Vaccinations." CNBC, August 30, 2021. https://www.cnbc.com/2021/08/30/krispy-kreme-doubles-its-free-doughnut-incentive-for-vaccinations.html

Dong, Yuanyuan, Xi Mo, Xin Qi, Fan Jiang, Zhongyi Jiang, and Shilu Tong. "Epidemiology of COVID-19 among Children in China." *Pediatrics* 2020;145(6):e20200702

Doshi, Peter. "Will Covid-19 Vaccines Save Lives? Current Trials Aren't Designed to Tell Us." *BMJ* 2020;371:m4037

Doshi, Peter. "Pfizer and Moderna's '95% Effective' Vaccines—Let's Be Cautious and First See the Full Data." *BMJ Blogs*, November 26, 2020. https://blogs.bmj.com/bmj/2020/11/26/peter-doshi-pfizer-and-modernas-95-effective-vaccines-lets-be-cautious-and-first-see-the-full-data/

Doshi, Peter. "Pfizer and Moderna's '95% Effective' Vaccines—We Need More Details and the Raw Data." *BMJ Blogs*, January 4, 2021. https://blogs.bmj.

com/bmj/2021/01/04/peter-doshi-pfizer-and-modernas-95-effective-vaccines-we-need-more-details-and-the-raw-data/

Doshi, Peter. "Covid-19 Vaccines in Children: Be Careful." UMB Digital Archives, June 10, 2021. https://archive.hshsl.umaryland.edu/handle/10713/16065

Doshi, Peter. "Does the FDA Think These Data Justify the First Full Approval of a COVID-19 Vaccine?" *BMJ Blogs*, August 23, 2021. https://blogs.bmj.com/bmj/2021/08/23/does-the-fda-think-these-data-justify-the-first-full-approval-of-a-covid-19-vaccine/

Doshi, Peter, Kay Dickersin, David Healy, S. Swaroop Vedula, and Tom Jefferson. "Restoring Invisible and Abandoned Trials: A Call for People to Publish the Findings." *BMJ* 2013;346:f2865

Doshi, Peter, Fiona Goodlee, and Kamran Abbasi. "Covid-19 Vaccines and Treatments: We Must Have Raw Data, Now." *BMJ* 2022;376:o102

Dudley, Sheldon F. "The Control of Diphtheria in Crowded Institutions." *Public Health* 42, (November 1928): 48-54.

Dudley, Sheldon F. "The Ecological Outlook on Epidemiology." *Proceedings of the Royal Society of Medicine* 30, no. 1 (1936): 57-70.

Dunn, Andrew. "A Coalition Backed by Bill Gates Is Funding Biotechs That Are Scrambling to Develop Vaccines for the Deadly Wuhan Cornonavirus." *Business Insider India*, January 23, 2020. https://www.businessinsider.in/science/news/a_coalition_backed_by_bill_gates_is_funding_biotechs_that_are_scrambling_to_develop_vaccines_for_the_deadly_wuhan_cornonavirus/articleshow/73559156.cms

Dyer, Evan. "Public Outrage over the Unvaccinated is Driving a Crisis in Bioethics." CBC News, January 22, 2022. https://www.cbc.ca/news/politics/pandemic-covid-vaccine-triage-omicron-1.6319844

Edelman, Alison, Emily R. Boniface, Victoria Male, Sharon T. Cameron, Eleonora Benhar, Leo Han, Kristan A. Matteson, Agathe Van Lamsweerde, Jack T. Pearson, and Blair G. Darney. "Association between Menstrual Cycle Length and Covid-19 Vaccination: Global, Retrospective Cohort Study of Prospectively Collected Data." *BMJMED* 2022;1:e000297

Edwards, Jim. "Blue Cross Names and Shames Pfizer Execs Linked to Massages-for-Prescriptions Push." CBS News, June 10, 2010. https://www.cbsnews.com/news/blue-cross-names-and-shames-pfizer-execs-linked-to-massages-for-prescriptions-push/

Elijah, Sonja. "Was Pfizer's 95% Vaccine Efficacy Fraudulent All Along?" Substack, April 3, 2022. https://soniaelijah.substack.com/p/was-pfizers-95-vaccine-efficacy-fraudulent?s=r

Eroshenko, Nikolai, Taylor Gill, Marianna K. Keaveny, George M. Church, Jose M. Trevejo, and Hannu Rajaniemi. "Implications of Antibody-Dependent Enhancement of Infection for SARS-CoV-2 Countermeasures." *Nature Biotechnology* 38, (July 2020): 788-797. https://doi.org/10.1038/s41587-020-0577-1

European Centre for Disease Prevention and Control. "COVID-19 in Children and the Role of School in Transmission—Second Update." July 8, 2021. https://www.ecdc.europa.eu/en/publications-data/children-and-school-settings-covid-19-transmission

European Medicines Agency. "EMA Recommends First COVID-19 Vaccine for Authorisation in the EU." December 12, 2020. https://www.ema.europa.eu/en/news/ema-recommends-first-covid-19-vaccine-authorisation-eu

Evans, Ryan. "Coronavirus Outbreak: 22 Deaths at Pemberley House Care Home." *Gazette*, January 27, 2021. https://www.basingstokegazette.co.uk/news/19043790.coronavirus-outbreak-22-deaths-pemberley-house-care-home/

Express Scripts. "America's State of Mind: US Trends in Medication Use for Depression, Anxiety, and Insomnia." April 2020. https://corporate-site-labs-prod.s3.us-east-2.amazonaws.com/2020-04/Express%20Scripts%20America%27s%20State%20of%20Mind%20Report%20April%202020%20FINAL_1.pdf

FDA. "Psychopharmacological Drugs Advisory Committee: Thirty-Third Meeting." 9:00 AM Monday, November 19, 1990.

FDA. "FDA Drug Safety Communication: FDA Updates Label for Stop Smoking Drug Chantix (Varenicline) to Include Potential Alcohol Interaction, Rare Risk of Seizures, and Studies of Side Effects on Mood, Behavior, or Thinking." March 9, 2015. https://www.fda.gov/drugs/drug-safe-ty-and-availability/fda-drug-safety-communication-fda-updates-la-bel-stop-smoking-drug-chantix-varenicline-include

FDA. "FDA Drug Safety Communication: FDA Revises Description of Mental Health Side Effects of the Stop-Smoking Medicines Chantix (Varenicline) and Zyban (Bupropion) to Reflect Clinical Trial Findings." December 16, 2016. https://www.fda.gov/drugs/drug-safety-and-avail-ability/fda-drug-safety-communication-fda-revises-description-men-tal-health-side-effects-stop-smoking

FDA. "What Is Gene Therapy?" July 25, 2018. https://www.fda.gov/vaccines-blood biologics/cellular-gene-therapy-products/what-gene-therapy

FDA. "FDA Takes Key Action in Fight against COVID-19 by Issuing Emergency Use Authorization for the First COVID-19 Vaccine." December 11, 2020. https://www.fda.gov/news-events/press-announce-ments/fda-takes-key-action-fight-against-covid-19-issuing-emergency-use-authorization-first-covid-19

FDA. "FDA Approves First Covid-19 Vaccine." August 23, 2021. https://www.fda.gov/news events/press-announcements/fda-approves-first-covid-19-vac-cine

FDA. "FDA Authorizes Booster Dose of Pfizer-BioNTech COVID-19 Vaccine for Certain Populations." September 22, 2021. https://www.fda.gov/news-events/press-announcements/fda-authorizes-booster-dose-pfizer-bi-ontech-covid-19-vaccine-certain-populations

FDA. "Coronavirus (COVID-19) Update: FDA Takes Additional Actions on the Use of a Booster Dose for COVID-19 Vaccine." October 20, 2021. https://www.fda.gov/news-events/press-announcements/coronavirus-covid-19-update-fda-takes-additional-actions-use-booster-dose-covid-19-vac-cines

FDA. "Vaccines and Related Biological Products Advisory Committee Meeting." October 26, 2021.

FDA. "Vaccines and Related Biological Products Advisory Committee—10/26/2021." YouTube, October 26, 2021. https://www.youtube.com/watch?v=laaL0_xKmmA&t=24733s

FDA. "FDA Authorizes Pfizer-BioNTech COVID-19 Vaccine for Emergency Use in Children 5 Through 11 Years of Age." October 29, 2021. https://www.fda.gov/news-events/press-announcements/fda-authorizes-pfizer-biontech-covid-19-vaccine-emergency-use-children-5-through-11-years-age

FDA. "Coronavirus (COVID-19) Update: FDA Authorizes Moderna, Pfizer-BioNTech COVID 19 Vaccines for Use as a Booster Dose." August 31, 2022.

FAIR Health. "Risk Factors for COVID-19 Mortality among Privately Insured Patients." November 11, 2020. https://www.fairhealth.org/publications/whitepapers

Fitzsimmons, Emma G. "Nearly 3,000 NYC Workers Have a Day to Get Vaccinated or Be Fired." *New York Times*, February 11, 2022.

Federal Emergency Management Agency. "Funeral Assistance FAQ." July 20, 2021. https://www.fema.gov/disaster/coronavirus/economic/funeral-assistance/faq

Florida Health. "Guidance for mRNA COVID-19 Vaccines." October 7, 2022.

Follmann, Dean, Holly E. James, Olive D. Buhle, Honghong Zhou, Bethany Girard, Kristen Marks, Karen Kotoloff, et al. "Anti-Nucleocapsid Antibodies following SARS-CoV-2 Infection in the Blinded Phase of the mRNA-1273 Covid-19 Vaccine Efficacy Clinical Trial." medRxiv preprint, April 19, 2022. https://www.medrxiv.org/content/10.1101/2022.04.18.22271936v1

Fox News. "Trudeau Has Lost Control of the Situation: Canadian Parliament Member." February 17, 2022. https://www.youtube.com/watch?v=ooi9rf-FUcic

Fraiman, Joseph, Juan Erviti, Mark Jones, Sander Greenland, Patrick Whelan, Robert M. Kaplan, and Peter Doshi. "Serious Adverse Events of Special Interest following mRNA COVID-19 Vaccination in Randomized Trials in Adults." *Vaccine* 40, no. 40 (September 22, 2022): 5798-5805. https://doi.org/10.1016/j.vaccine.2022.08.036

Garde, Damian. "Sanofi Inks a $1.5B Deal to Join BioNTech's Growing List of Oncology Partners." *Fierce Biotech*, November 3, 2015. https://www.

fiercebiotech.com/partnering/sanofi-inks-a-1-5b-deal-to-join-biontech-s-growing-list-of-oncology-partners

Garde, Damian. "Ego, Ambition, and Turmoil: Inside One of Biotech's Most Secretive Startups." *STAT*, September 13, 2016. https://www.statnews.com/2016/09/13/moderna-therapeutics-biotech-mrna/

Garde, Damian. "Lavishly Funded Moderna Hits Safety Problems in Bold Bid to Revolutionize Medicine." *STAT*, January 10, 2017. https://www.statnews.com/2017/01/10/moderna-trouble-mrna/

Gardiner, Harris. "Pfizer to Pay $2.3 Billion to Settle Inquiry over Marketing." *New York Times*, September 3, 2009, B4.

Gardiner, Harris, and Duff Wilson. "FDA Warns of Side Effects for 2 Stop-Smoking Drugs." *New York Times*, July 2, 2009, B2.

Garner, Paul. "For Seven Weeks I Have Been Through a Roller Coaster of Ill Health, Extreme Emotions, and Utter Exhaustion." *BMJ Blogs*, May 5, 2020. https://blogs.bmj.com/bmj/2020/05/05/paul-garner-people-who-have-a-more-protracted-illness-need-help-to-understand-and-cope-with-the-constantly-shifting-bizarre-symptoms/

Gates, Bill. "Here Are the Innovations We Need to Reopen the Economy." *Washington Post*, April 23, 2020. https://www.washingtonpost.com/opinions/2020/04/23/bill-gates-here-are-innovations-we-need-reopen-economy/

Gazit, Sivan, Roef Shlezinger, Galit Perez, Roni Lotan, Asaf Peretz, Amir Ben-Tov, Dani Cohen, Khitam Muhsen, Gabriel Chodick, and Tal Patalon. "Comparing SARS-CoV-2 Natural Immunity to Vaccine-Induced Immunity: Reinfections versus Breakthrough Infections." medRxiv preprint, August 25, 2021. https://doi.org10.1101/2021.08.24.21262415

Goldberg, Yair, Micha Mandel, Yinon M. Bar-On, Orriri Bodenheimer, Laurence Freedman, Eric J. Haas, Ron Milo, Sharon Alroy-Preis, Nachman Ash, and Amit Huppert. "Waning Immunity after the BNT162b Vaccine in Israel." *New England Journal of Medicine* 385, no. 4 (December 9, 2021). https:doi.org/10.1056/NEJMoa2114228

Goodlee, Fiona, and Kamran Abbasi. "Open Letter to Mark Zuckerberg." *BMJ*, December 17, 2021. https://www.bmj.com/content/375/bmj.n2635/rr-80

Gorski, David. "COVID-19 Deniers Follow the Path Laid Down by Creationists, HIV/AIDS Denialists, and Climate Science Deniers." Science-Based Medicine, October 12, 2020. https://sciencebasedmedicine.org/great-barrington-declaration/

Gorski, David. "Why Is Peter Doshi Still an Editor at the BMJ?" Respectful Insolence, January 15, 2021. https://respectfulinsolence.com/2021/01/15/why-is-peter-doshi-still-an-editor-at-the-bmj/

Gorski, David. "The '12% Efficacy' Myth from the 'Pfizer Data Dump': The Latest Slasher Stat about COVID-19 Vaccines." Science-Based Medicine, May 9, 2022. https://sciencebasedmedicine.org/the-12-gambit-the-latest-slasher-stat-about-covid-19-vaccines/

Gorski, David. "The State of Florida Spreads Antivaccine Disinformation Disguised as an Epidemiological Study." Science-Based Medicine, October 10, 2022. https://sciencebasedmedicine.org/the-state-of-florida-spreads-antivaccine-disinformation-disguised-as-an-epidemiological-study/

Grady, Denise. "Testing on Humans Begins for an Experimental Vaccine." *New York Times*, March 17, 2020, A12.

Grady, Denise, and Katie Thomas. "2 Firms Share Plans on Trials for a Vaccine." *New York Times*, September 18, 2020, A1.

Greene, Jenna. "Wait What? FDA Wants 55 Years to Process FOIA Request over Vaccine Data." Reuters, November 18, 2021. https://www.reuters.com/legal/government/wait-what-fda-wants-55-years-process-foia-request-over-vaccine-data-2021-11-18/

Greene, Jenna. "We'll All Be Dead Before FDA Releases Full Covid Vaccine Records, Plaintiffs Say." Reuters, December 14, 2021. https://www.reuters.com/legal/government/well-all-be-dead-before-fda-releases-full-covid-vaccine-record-plaintiffs-say-2021-12-13/

Griffin, Drew, and Andy Segal. "Feds Found Pfizer Too Big to Nail." CNN, April 2, 2010. http://www.cnn.com/2010/HEALTH/04/02/pfizer.bextra/index.html

Grimes, Katy. "California Doctors Sue Gov. Newsom and Medical Board over New Law Censoring Medical Advice." *California Globe*, November 2, 2022.

https://californiaglobe.com/articles/california-doctors-sue-gov-newsom-and-medical-board-over-new-law-censoring-medical-advice/

HART Group. "Only a Fraction of the Population is Susceptible to Each Variant." December 9, 2021. https://www.hartgroup.org/only-a-fraction-of-the-population-are-susceptible-to-each-variant/

HART Group. "Where's the Evidence for Waning Vaccine Immunity?" February 17, 2022. https://www.hartgroup.org/wheres-the-evidence-for-waning-vaccine-immunity/

Hansen, Christian Holm, Astrid Blicher Schelde, Ida Rask Moustsen-Helm, Hanne-Dorthe Emborg, Tyra, Kåre Mølbak, and Palle Valentiner-Branth. "Vaccine Effectiveness against SARS-CoV-2 Infection with the Omicron or Delta Variants Following a Two-Dose or Booster BNT162b2 mRNA Vaccination Series: A Danish Cohort Study." medRxiv preprint, December 22, 2021. https://www.medrxiv.org/content/10.1101/2021.12.20.21267966v2

Haroun, Azmi, and Hilary Bruek. "CDC Director Says Data 'Suggests That Vaccinated People Do Not Carry the Virus.'" *Business Insider,* March 30, 2021. https://www.businessinsider.com/cdc-director-data-vaccinated-people-do-not-carry-covid-19-2021-3

Harper, Phil. "A Public Verification of Jikkyleaks." Substack, June 8, 2022. https://philharper.substack.com/p/a-public-verification-of-jikkyleaks

Hauser, Chris. "Get a COVID-19 Vaccine or Face Prison, Judges Order in Probation Cases." *New York Times*, August 9, 2021.

Healy, David. *Pharmageddon*. Berkeley, California: University of California Press, March 12, 2012.

Healy, David. "Report Covid Vaccine Effects to RxISK." RxISK, January 11, 2021. https://rxisk.org/report-covid-vaccine-effects-to-rxisk/

Healy, David. "A Reason for Hesitancy." *BMJ*, December 27, 2021. https://www.bmj.com/content/375/bmj.n3152/rr

Healy, David. "The Evidence That Counts for the FDA." January 19, 2022. https://davidhealy.org/the-evidence-that-counts-for-fda/

Healy, David. "The Evidence That Counts for Us." January 26, 2022. https://davidhealy.org/the-evidence-that-counts-for-us/

Healy, David. "The Crack through Which Science Gets in." February 15, 2022. https://davidhealy.org/the-crack-through-which-the-science-gets-in/

Healy, David. "Injuries in Vaccine Trials." February 22, 2022. https://davidhealy.org/injuries-in-vaccine-trials/

Healy, David, Joann LeNoury, and Julie Wood. *Children of the Cure: Missing Data, Lost Lives, and Antidepressants.* Toronto: Samizdat Health Writer's Co-operative, 2020.

Healy, Melissa. "Are the Unvaccinated Still a Danger to the Rest of Us?" *Los Angeles Times*, November 3, 2022.

Hensley, Scott. "Pfizer Makes Aid Pledge, Breaks Aid Pact." *Wall Street Journal*, November 12, 2003, B1.

Hernandez, Joe. "Nearly 94,000 Kids Got COVID-19 Last Week. They Were 15% of All New Cases." National Public Radio, August 10, 2021. https://www.npr.org/sections/coronavirus-live-updates/2021/08/10/1026375608/nearly-94-000-kids-got-covid-19-last-week-they-were-15-of-all-new-infections

Herper, Matthew. "Bextra! Bextra! Pharmacia Drug Approved!" *Forbes*, November 19, 2001. https://www.forbes.com/2001/11/19/1119bextra.html?sh=13d6b04f11ee

Herper, Matthew. "Can Chantix Make a Comeback?" *Forbes*, September 12, 2008. https://www.forbes.com/2008/09/11/pfizer-smoking-chantix-biz-healthcare-cx_mh_0911chantix.html?sh=2f3d36be6d95

Hiltzik, Michael. "Mocking Anti-Vaxxers' Covid Deaths Is Ghoulish, Yes—But May Be Necessary." *Los Angeles Times*, January 10, 2022.

Hoffman, Jan. "Few Parents Say They Plan to Vaccinate Young Children against Covid." *New York Times*, July 27, 2022, A17.

Holan, Angie Drobnic. "Poynter Institute Announces Initiative to Fact-Check Claims about Global Health and Development." PolitiFact, January 25, 2016. https://www.politifact.com/artice/2016/jan/25/poynter-institute-announces-initiative-fact-check-/

Hooker, Lucy, and Daniele Palumbo. "Covid Vaccines: Will Drug Companies Make Bumper Profits?" BBC Business, December 18, 2020. https://www.bbc.com/news/business-55170756

Huang, Chaolin, Yeming Wang, Xingwang Li, Lili Ren, Jianping Zhou, Yi Hu, Li Zhang, et al. "Clinical Features of Patients Infected with 2019 Novel Coronavirus in Wuhan, China." *Lancet* 395, no. 10223 (February 15, 2020): 497-506. https://doi.org/10.1016/S0140-6736(20)30183-5

Hudson, Polly. "As Covid Restrictions Ease, It's Time to Get Tough on Anti-Vaxxers." *Mirror*, January 25, 2022. https://www.mirror.co.uk/news/uk-news/as-covid-restrictions-ease-its-26046616?fbclid=IwAR30KhFu-rOXa4sE0l79TBPPfL5lJLZ9JylvUShS5daW_wHciLkYqcIR14ak

Hunter, Paul, and Julii Brainard. "Estimating the Effectiveness of the Pfizer COVID-19, BNT162b2 Vaccine after a Single Dose. A Reanalysis of a Study of 'Real-World' Vaccination Outcomes from Israel." medRxiv preprint, February 3, 2021. https://www.medrxiv.org/content/10.1101/2021.02.01.21250957v1

i24NEWS. "Vaccine 39% Effective at Halting Virus Transmission, 91% against Serious Illness, Israel's Health Ministry Says." July 22, 2021. https://www.i24news.tv/en/news/coronavirus/1626980447-vaccine-39-effective-at-halting-virus-transmission-91-against-serious-illness-israel-s-health-ministry-says

i24NEWS. "This is Not the Time to Debate Vaccines but to Get Them, Israel's Bennett Tells Refusniks." July 22, 2021. https://www.i24news.tv/en/news/israel/1626976195-this-is-not-the-time-to-debate-vaccines-but-to-get-them-israel-s-bennett-tells-refuseniks

Iacobucci, Gareth. "Covid-19: FDA Set to Grant Full Approval to Pfizer Vaccine without Public Discussion of Data." *BMJ* 2021;374n2086

Internet Archive Wayback Machine. "Vaccine." November 5, 2020. https://web.archive.org/web/20201105154809/https://www.merriam-webster.com/dictionary/vaccine

Jaafar, Rita, Sarah Aherfi, Nathalie Wurtz, Clio Grimaldier, Thuan Van Hoang, Phillipe Colson, Didier Raoult, and Bernard La Scola. "Correlation between 3790 Quantitative Polymerase Chain Reaction-Positive Samples and Positive Cell Cultures, Including 1941 Severe Acute Respiratory Syndrome Coronavirus 2 Isolates." *Clinical Infectious Diseases* 72, no. 11 (June 1, 2021): e921. https://doi.org/10.1093/ciaa1491

Jenner, Edward. *An Inquiry into the Causes and Effects of the Variole Vaccinae, or Cow-Pox*. London: Sampson and Low, 1798.

Jiménez, Jesus. "Washington State Allows for Free Marijuana with COVID-19 Vaccine." *New York Times*, June 7, 2021.

Johnson, Raymond M., Peter Doshi, and David Healy. "Covid-19: Should Doctors Recommend Treatments and Vaccines When Full Data Are Not Publicly Available?" *BMJ* 2020;370:m3260

Joyella, Mark. "CNN's Don Lemon on the Unvaccinated: 'Their Behavior Is Idiotic and Nonsensical.'" *Forbes*, July 24, 2021. https://www.forbes.com/sites/markjoyella/2021/07/24/cnns-don-lemon-on-the-unvaccinated-their-behavior-is-idiotic-and-nonsensical/?sh=752cd52f4b76

Kanduc, Darja. "Peptide Cross-Reactivity: The Original Sin of Vaccines." *Frontiers in Bioscience* S4, (June 1, 2021): 1393-1401. https://doi.org/10.2741/s341 Kanduc, Darja, and Yehuda Schoenfeld. "Molecular Mimicry between SARS-CoV-2 Spike

Glycoprotein and Mammalian Proteomes: Implications for the Vaccine." *Immunologic Research* 68, no. 5 (2020): 310-313. https://doi.org/1007/s12026-020-09152-6

Kanno-Youngs, Zolan, and Cecilia Kang. "'They're Killing People': Biden Denounces Social Media for Virus Disinformation." *New York Times*, July 16, 2021.

Kansas State Agricultural College Experimental Station. "Contagious Abortion of Cattle." August 1918.

Kaplan, Shelia. "Hahn Leaves FDA; Woodcock Named Acting Commissioner." *New York Times*, January 20, 2021.

Keay, Lara. "Long-Term Covid Warning: ICU Doctor Reports Having Coronavirus Symptoms for Three Months." Sky News, June 25, 2020. https://news.sky.com/story/long-term-covid-warning-icu-doctor-reports-having-coronavirus-symptoms-for-three-months-12014361

Kenealy, Edel. "Scots Care Home Residents Test Positive for Covid-19 Days after Receiving Vaccine." *Daily Record*, January 6, 2021. https://www.dailyrecord.co.uk/news/local-news/care-home-residents-test-positive-23269764

Kershner, Isabel. "Israel's Push to Vaccinate Raises Host of Legal, Moral and Ethical Questions." *New York Times*, February 19, 2021, A6.

Kheriaty, Aaron. "Our Lawsuit Uncovers Army of Federal Bureaucrats Coercing Social-Media Companies to Censor Speech." Substack, September 1, 2022. https://aaronkheriaty.substack.com/p/our-lawsuit-uncovers-army-of-federal

Kime, Patricia. "Pentagon Tracking 14 Cases of Heart Inflammation in Troops after COVID-19 Shots." military.com, April 26, 2021. https://www.military.com/daily-news/2021/04/26/pentagon-tracking-14-cases-of-heart-inflam-mation-troops-after-covid-19-shots.html

Kochi, Sudiksha. "Fact Check: Missing Context in Claim That Merriam-Webster Changed 'Vaccine' Definition." *USA Today*, November 30, 2021. https://www.usatoday.com/story/news/factcheck/2021/11/30/fact-check-merri-am-webster-changed-vaccine-definition-accuracy/6354415001/

Kochi, Sudiksha. "Fact Check: Claim Misrepresents Data from a Pfizer 2021 Report." *USA Today*, May 30, 2022. https://www.usatoday.com/story/news/factcheck/2022/05/30/fact-check-claim-misinterprets-data-2021-pfizer-re-port/9898129002/

Kojima, Noah, and Jeffrey D. Klausner. "Protective Immunity after Recovery from SARS-CoV 2 Infection." *Lancet Infectious Diseases* 22, no. 1 (January 2022): 12-14. https://doi.org/10.1016/S1473-3099(21)00676-9

Kornick, Lindsay. "Liberals Cheer on Biden's Anger toward the Unvaccinated During Covid Address." Fox News, September 9, 2021. https://www.foxnews.com/media/intense-mixed-reactions-biden-anger-at-the-unvacci-nated

Krause, Philip R., and Luciana Borio. "The Biden Administration Has Been Sidelining Vaccine Experts." *Washington Post*, December 19, 2021, B2.

Kranjec, Jastra. "Pfizer-BioNTech and Moderna to Earn $14.7 B in COVID 19 Vaccine Sales by 2023." Finaria, January 19, 2021. https://www.finaria.it/pr/pfizer-biontech-and-moderna-to-earn-14-7b-from-covid-19-vaccines-sales-by-2023/

Krepps, Daniel. "Howard Stern to 'Imbecile' Anti-Vaxxers: 'Go F—k Yourself.'" *Rolling Stone*, September 9, 2021. https://www.rollingstone.com/culture/culture-news/howard-stern-anti-vaxxers-go-fuck-yourself-1222672/

Kulldorff, Martin, Sunetra Gupta, and Jay Bhattacharya. "Great Barrington Declaration." October 4, 2020. https://gbdeclaration.org/

La Scola, Bernard, Marion Le Bideau, Julien Andreani, Van Thuan Hoang, Clio Grimaldier, Phillipe Colson, Phillipe Gautret, and Didier Raoult. "Viral RNA Load as Determined by Cell Culture as a Management Tool for Discharge of SARS-CoV-2 Patients from Infectious Disease Wards." *European Journal of Clinical Microbiology and Infectious Diseases* 39, no. 6 (June 2020): 1059-1061. https://doi.org/10.1007/s10096-020-03913-9

LaFraniere, Sharon, and Noah Weiland. "Pfizer Asks FDA to Clear 2 Vaccine Doses for Young Children as a Start." *New York Times*, February 1, 2022, A10.

LaFraniere, Sharon, and Noah Weiland. "FDA Delays Shots for Those Under Age of 5." *New York Times*, February 12, 2022, A1.

LaFraniere, Sharon. "FDA May Move toward Updating Vaccines." *New York Times*, June 27, 2022.

Lahucik, Kyle. "He Authorized Moderna's Vaccine 6 Months Ago. Now Ex-FDA Chief Hahn Joins Biotech's Backer." *Fierce Biotech*, July 14, 2021. https://www.fiercebiotech.com/biotech/six-months-after-granting-moderna-covid-19-eua-ex-fda-commish-joins-biotech-s-founding

Lavine, Jennie S., Ottar Bjornstadt, and Rustom Antia. "Vaccinating Children against SARS-CoV-2." *BMJ* 2021;373n117

Leatherby, Lauren. "How the BA.5 Subvariant May Affect the US." *New York Times*, July 8, 2022, A11.

Lee, Katherine M.N., Eleanor J. Junkins, Urooba A. Fatima, Maria L. Cox, and Kathryn B.H. Clancy. "Characterizing Menstrual Bleeding Changes Occurring after SARS-CoV-2 Vaccination." medRxiv preprint, October 12, 2021. https://www.medrxiv.org/content/10.1101/2021.10.11.21264863v1

Lemon, Jason. "Video of Biden Saying Vaccinations Prevent Covid Resurfaces after Infection." *Newsweek*, July 21, 2022. https://www.newsweek.com/joe-biden-2021-video-saying-vaccinations-prevent-covid-resurfaces-1726900

Letcher, Lisa. "Eleven Residents Die in Three Weeks after Care Home Covid Outbreak." CornwallLive, February 15, 2021. https://www.cornwalllive. com/news/cornwall-news/eleven-residents-die-three-weeks-5005443

Li, Bo, Jing Yang, Faming Zhao, Lili Zhi, Xiqian Wang, Lin Liu, Zhaohui Bi, and Yunhe Zhao. "Prevalence and Impact of Cardiovascular Metabolic Diseases on COVID-19 in China." *Clinical Research in Cardiology* 109, no. 5 (May 2020): 531-538. https://doi.org/10.1007/s00392-020-01626-9

Lin II, Rong-Gong. "Fears of More Long Covid, a 'Mass Disabling Event' as Variants Rip Through California." *Los Angeles Times*, July 26, 2022. https:// www.latimes.com/california/story/2022-07-26/covid-19-reinfection-wors- ens-long-term-risk-for-death-fatigue-heart-disorders

Lovelace, Berkely. "CDC OKs Pfizer's Covid Vaccine for Use in Adolescents, Clearing the Way for Shots to Begin Thursday." CNBC, May 12, 2021. https://www.cnbc.com/2021/05/12/pfizer-covid-vaccine-cdc-panel-endors- es-for-use-in-kids-12-to-15.html

Lowe, Derek. "Spike Protein Behavior." *Science Blogs*, May 4, 2021. https://www. science.org/content/blog-post/spike-protein-behavior

MSNBC. "Transcript: All in One with Chris Hayes, 5/17/21." May 17, 2021. https://www.msnbc.com/transcripts/transcript-all-chris-hayes-5-17- 21-n1267740

MacArthur, John R. "The Publisher's Role: Crusading Defender of the First Amendment or Advertising Salesman?" In *The Art of Making Magazines: On Being an Editor and Other Views from the Industry*, edited by Victor S. Navasky and Evan Cornog, 141-153. New York: Columbia University Press, 2012.

Mahase, Elizabeth. "Covid-19: What Do We Know About 'Long Covid?'" *BMJ* 2020;370:m2815

Mallick, Heather. "The Unvaccinated Cherish Their Freedom to Harm Others. How Can We Ever Forgive Them?" *Toronto Star*, January 15, 2022. https:// www.thestar.com/politics/political-opinion/2022/01/15/the-unvaccinated- cherish-their-freedom-to-harm-others-how-can-we-ever-forgive-them. html

Malloy, Allie, and Maegan Vazquez. "Biden Warns of Winter of 'Severe Illness and Death' for Unvaccinated Due to Omicron." CNN, December 16, 2021. https://www.cnn.com/2021/12/16/politics/joe-biden-warning-winter/index. html

Malone, Robert W., Phillip L. Felgner, and Inder M. Verma. "Cationic Liposome-Mediated RNA Transfection." *Proceedings of the National Academy of Sciences* 86, no. 16 (August 1989): 6077-6081. https://doi. org/10.1073/pnas.86/16/6077

Mandavilli, Apoorva. "Your Coronavirus Test Is Positive. Maybe It Shouldn't Be." *New York Times*, August 29, 2020.

Mandavilli, Apoorva. "CDC Data Suggests Boosters' Protection against Severe COVID-19 Plunges after 4 Months." *New York Times*, February 11, 2022.

Mandavilli, Apoorva. "CDC Isn't Publishing Large Portion of COVID-19 Data It Collects." *New York Times*, February 20, 2022.

Mandavilli, Apoorva. "As Vaccines Arrive for the Youngest, Parents are Put on the Spot." *New York Times*, June 19, 2022, A1.

Mandavilli, Apoorva. "Will Covid Boosters Prevents Another Wave? Scientists Aren't So Sure." *New York Times*, November 19, 2022.

Massetti, Greta, Brendan R. Jackson, John T. Brooks, Cria G. Perrine, Erica Reott, Aron J. Hall, Debra Lubar, et al. "Summary of Guidance for Minimizing the Impact of COVID-19 in Individual Persons, Communities, and Health Care Systems—United States, August 2022." *Morbidity and Mortality Weekly Report* 71, (August 11, 2022): 1-9. https://www.cdc.gov/ mmwr/volumes/71/wr/mm7133e1.htm

Mathioudakis, Alexander G., Murad Ghrew, Andrew Ustianowski, Shazaad Ahmad, Ray Borrow, Lida Pieretta Papavasileoui, Dimitrios Petrakis, and Nawar Diar Bakerly. "Self-Reported Real-World Safety and Reactogenicity of COVID-19 Vaccines: A Vaccine Recipient Survey." *Life*, 11, no. 249 (2021): 1-13. https://doi.org/10.3390/life11030249

McAuley, James. "Macron is Right: It's Time to Make Life a Living Hell for Anti-Vaxxers." *Washington Post*, January 11, 2022.

McCutchan, Ellen. "Viral Pfizer 'Admission' Not What It Seems." RMIT FactLab, November 3, 2022. https://www.rmit.edu.au/news/factlab-meta/viral-pfizer--admission--not-what-it-seems?fbclid=IwAR2Xjry-TOddm9-ihUIyR17Suw8zbKCJ0qWA-9Zn0J3M7i7ssiLUOqYzVau0

McElvoy, Anne. "The Unvaccinated Have Become a Lethal Liability We Can Ill-Afford." *Evening Standard*, December 14, 2021. https://www.standard.co.uk/comment/covid-unvaccinated-omicron-vaccine-passports-b971877.html

McNeil, Donald G. "How Much Herd Immunity Is Enough?" *New York Times,* December 24, 2020.

Menge, Margaret. "Indiana Life Insurance CEO Says Deaths Are up 40% among People Ages 18-64." Center Square, January 1, 2022. https://www.thecentersquare.com/indiana/indiana-life-insurance-ceo-says-deaths-are-up-40-among-people-ages-18-64/article_71473b12-6b1e-11ec-8641-5b2c06725e2c.html

Merlan, Anna. "Anti-Vaxxers are Terrified the Government Will Enforce a Vaccine for Coronavirus." *Vice*, February 28, 2020. https://www.vice.com/en/article/m7q5vv/anti-vaxxers-are-terrified-the-government-will-enforce-a-vaccine-for-coronavirus

Merriam-Webster. "Vaccine." Accessed May 17, 2022. https://www.merriam webster.com/dictionary/vaccine

Miller, Dean. "Fact Check: The BMJ Did NOT Reveal Disqualifying and Ignored Reports of Flaws in Pfizer COVID-19 Vaccine Trials." Lead Stories, November 10, 2021. https://leadstories.com/hoax-alert/2021/11/fact-check-british-medical-journal-did-not-reveal-disqualifying-and-ignored-reports-of-flaws-in-pfizer-vaccine-trial.html

Miller, Dean. "Lead Stories Response to BMJ Open Letter Objecting to a Lead Stories Fact Check." Lead Stories, December 18, 2021. https://leadstories.com/analysis/2021/12/lead-stories-response-to-a-bmjcom-open-letter-objecting-to-a-lead-stories-fact-check.html

Miller, Megan. "Lawsuit Claims Economy Murder-Suicide Caused by Stop-Smoking Drug." *Star-Courier*, May 9, 2011. https://www.starcourier.

com/story/news/crime/2011/05/10/lawsuit-claims-economy-murder-sui-
cide/18379085007/

Misra, Puneet, Shashi Kant, Randeep Guleria, Sanjay K. Rai, and the WHO
Unity Seroprevalence Study Team of AIIMS. "Serological Prevalence of
SARS-CoV-2 Antibody among Children and Young Age (Between Age
2-17 Years) Group in India: An Interim Result from a Large Multicentric
Population-Based Seroepidemiological Study." medRxiv preprint, June 16,
2021. https://www.medrxiv.org/content/10.1101/2021.06.15.21258880v1

Moderna. "A Phase 3, Randomized, Stratified, Observer-Blind, Placebo-Controlled Study to Evaluate the Efficacy, Safety, and Immunogenicity of
mRNA-1273 SARS-CoV-2 Vaccine in Adults Aged 18 Years and Older."
August 20, 2020. https://covid19crc.org/publications-and-resources/covid-
19-studies/moderna/

Moderna. "Moderna's COVID-19 Vaccine Candidate Meets Its Primary
Efficacy Endpoint in the First Interim Analysis of the Phase 3 COVE
Study." November 16, 2020. https://www.biospace.com/article/releases/
moderna-s-covid-19-vaccine-candidate-meets-its-primary-efficacy-end-
point-in-the-first-interim-analysis-of-the-phase-3-cove-study/

Moderna. "mRNA Platform: Enabling Drug Discovery and Development."
Accessed April 3, 2022. https://www.modernatx.com

Moderna. "Moderna Reports First Quarter 2022 Financial Results and Provides
Business Updates." May 4, 2022. https://investors.modernatx.com/news/
news-details/2022/Moderna-Reports-First-Quarter-2022-Financial-Res-
ults-and-Provides-Business-Updates/default.aspx

Montano, Diego. "Frequency and Associations of Adverse Reactions of
COVID-19 Vaccines Reported to Pharmacovigilance Systems in the
European Union and the United States." *Frontiers in Public Health*
9, Article 756633 (February 3, 2022): 1-16. https://doi.org/10.3389/
fpubh.2021.756633

Moore, Thomas J., Michael Cohen, and Curt D. Furberg. "Strong Safety Signal
Seen for Chantix (Varenicline)." *QuarterWatch*, May 25, 2008, 1-14.

Moore, Thomas J., Michael Cohen, and Curt D. Furberg. "Thoughts and Acts of
Aggression/Violence toward Others Reported in Association with Vareni-

cline." *Annals of Pharmacotherapy* 44, no. 9 (September 2010): 1389-1394. https://doi.org/10.1345/aph.1OP172

Moore, Thomas J., Michael Cohen, and Curt D. Furberg. "Prescription Drugs Associated with Reports of Violence towards Others." *PLoS One* 5, no. 12 (December 15, 2010). https://doi.org/10.1371/journal.pone.0015337

Moore, Thomas J., Michael Cohen, and Curt D. Furberg. "New Varenicline (CHANTIX) Suicide Cases." *QuarterWatch,* May 19, 2011, 2.

Moore, Thomas J., Michael Cohen, and Curt D. Furberg. "Varenicline (CHANTIX) and Suicidal/Homicidal Thoughts." *QuarterWatch*, September 24, 2014.

Morens, David M., Jeffrey K. Taubenberger, and Anthony S. Fauci. "Rethinking Next Generation Vaccines for Coronaviruses, Influenzaviruses, and Other Respiratory Diseases." *Cell Host & Microbe* 31, no. 1 (January 11, 2023): 146-157. https://doi.org/10.1016/chom.202211.06

Morris, Jeffrey. "Do the Recent 80k Pages of Pfizer Documents Released Really Show Vaccine Efficacy Was Only 12%?" Covid-19 Data Science, May 5, 2022. https://www.covid-datascience.com/post/do-the-recent-80k-pages-of-pfizer-documents-released-really-show-vaccine-efficacy-was-only-12

Moustsen-Helmes, Ida Rask, Hanne-Dorothe Emborg, Jens Nielsen, Katrine Finderup Nielsen, Tyra Grove, Kåre Mølbak, Karina Lauenborg Møller, Ann-Sofie Nicole Berthelsen, and Palle Valentiner-Branth. "Vaccine Effectiveness after 1st and 2nd Dose of the BNT162b2 mRNA COVID-19 Vaccine in Long-Term Care Facility Residents and Healthcare Workers—a Danish Cohort Study." medRxiv preprint, March 9, 2021. https://www.medrxiv.org/content/10.1101/2021.03.08.21252200v1

Mulligan, Mark J., Kirsten E. Lyke, Nicholas Kitchin, Judith Absalon, Alejandra Gurtman, Stephen Lockhart, Kathleen Neuzil, et al. "Phase I/II Study of COVID-19 RNA Vaccine BNT162b1 in Adults." *Nature* 586, (October 22, 2020): 589-593. https://doi.org/10.1038/s41586-020-2639-4

Muoio, David. "How Many Employees Have Hospitals Lost to Vaccine Mandates? Here Are the Numbers So Far." *Fierce Healthcare*, February 22, 2022. https://www.fiercehealthcare.com/hospitals/how-many-employees-have-hospitals-lost-to-vaccine-mandates-numbers-so-far

Musto, Julia. "CDC Director Rochelle Walensky Tests Positive for COVID-19 Month after Getting Updated Booster Shot." Fox News, October 22, 2022. https://www.foxnews.com/health/cdc-director-rochelle-walensky-tests-positive-covid-19-month-getting-updated-booster-shot

National Institute of Allergies and Infectious Disease. "NIH Clinical Trial of Investigational Vaccine for COVID-19 Begins." March 16, 2020. https://www.niaid.nih.gov/diseases-conditions/coronaviruses

National Institutes of Health. "Study Confirms Link Between COVID-19 Vaccination and Temporary Increase in Menstrual Cycle Length." September 27, 2022. https://www.nih.gov/news-events/news-releases/study-confirms-link-between-covid-19-vaccination-temporary-increase-menstrual-cycle-length

Nature. "What the Moderna-NIH Covid Vaccine Patent Fight Means for Research." November 30, 2021. https://doi.org/10.1038/d41586-021-03535-x

Naylor, Dave. "Trudeau Calls the Unvaccinated Racist and Misogynistic Extremists." *Western Standard News*, December 29, 2021. https://www.westernstandard.news/news/trudeau-calls-the-unvaccinated-racist-and-misogynistic-extremists/article_a3bacece-2e14-5b8c-bf37-eddd672205f3.html

Neil, Andrew. "It's Time to Punish Britain's Five Million Vaccine Refuseniks." *Daily Mail*, December 9, 2021. https://www.dailymail.co.uk/debate/article-10294225/Its-time-punish-Britains-five-million-vaccine-refuseniks-says-ANDREW-NEIL.html

New York City. "Mayor de Blasio Announces Vaccine Mandate for New York City Workers." October 20, 2021. https://www.nyc.gov/office-of-the-mayor/news/698-21/mayor-de-blasio-vaccine-mandate-new-york-city-workforce

New York City. "Mayor de Blasio Announces Vaccine Mandate for Private Sector Workers, and Major Expansions to Nation-Leading 'Key to NYC Program.'" December 6, 2021. https://www.nyc.gov/office-of-the-mayor/news/807-21/mayor-de-blasio-vaccine-mandate-private-sector-workers-major-expansions-to

New York Times. "Around the World." May 7, 2020, A12.

New York Times. "Pfizer Continues Spree with $5.4 Billion Buy." August 9, 2022, B2.

New Zealand Herald. "New Zealand Enters Nationwide Lockdown in Fight against COVID 19." March 25, 2020. https://nzhistory.govt.nz/page/new-zealand-enters-nationwide-lockdown-fight-against-covid-19

Ng, Kevin, Nikhil Faulkner, Georgina H. Cornish, Annachiara Rosa, Ruth Harvey, Saira Hussain, Rachel Ulferts, et al. "Serological Prevalence of SARS-CoV-2 Antibody among Children and Young Age (Between Age 2-17 Years) Group in India: An Interim Result from a Large Multicentric Population-Based Seroepidemiological Study." medRxiv preprint, June 16, 2021. https://www.medrxiv.org/content/10.1101/2021.06.15.21258880v1

Notheis, Asher. "Don Lemon Says Unvaccinated Should be 'Shunned' or 'Left behind.'" Yahoo News, September 16, 2021. https://www.yahoo.com/video/don-lemon-says-unvaccinated-people-175300636.html

Olive, David. "Vaccine Resisters Are Lazy and Irresponsible—We Need Vaccine Passports Now to Protect the Rest of Us." *Toronto Star*, July 30, 2021. https://www.thestar.com/business/opinion/2021/07/30/we-need-a-national-vaccination-passport-recognized-throughout-the-world.html

Oster, Emily. "Let's Declare a Pandemic Amnesty." *Atlantic*, October 31, 2022.

Palmer, Ewan. "What 'Pfizer Documents' Release Reveals." *Newsweek*, May 22, 2022. https://www.newsweek.com/pfizer-documents-vaccine-deaths-1703869

Pasteur, Louis. "Sur les Maladies Virulentes et en Particulier sur la Maladie Apellée Vulgairment Choléra des Poules." *Comptes Rendus Hemdomaires des Séances de l'Academie des Sciences* 90, (1880): 239-248.

Payne, Ed. "Fact Check: DOD Whistleblowers 'Mind Blowing Covid Vaccine Injury Numbers' Were Not Based on Accurate Data, Pentagon Says." Lead Stories, February 1, 2022. https://leadstories.com/hoax-alert/2022/02/fact-check-dod-whistleblowers-mind-blowing-covid-vaccine-injury-numbers-were-not-based-on-accurate-data.html?fbclid=IwAR05_--On8kEKHdfxSf130eN5J7sGY3AloIK3u3xCoVg0SZmWt6hz-9Rwbcs

Petersen, Melody. *Our Daily Meds*. New York: Sarah Crichton Books, 2008.

Pezenik, Sasha. "Alcohol Consumption Rising Sharply during Pandemic, Especially among Women." ABC News, September 29, 2020. https://abcnews.go.com/US/alcohol-consumption-rising-sharply-pandemic-women/story?id=73302479

Pfizer. "A Phase 1/2/3 Placebo-Controlled, Randomized, Observer-Blind Dose-Finding Study to Evaluate the Safety, Tolerability, Immunogenicity, and Efficacy of SARS-2-CoV RNA Vaccine Candidates against COVID-19 in Healthy Individuals." Accessed June 15, 2022. https://cdn.pfizer.com/pfizercom/2020-11/C4591001_Clinical_Protocol_Nov2020.pdf

Pfizer. "Pfizer and BioNTech Announce Vaccine Candidate against COVID-19 Achieved Success in First Interim Analysis from Phase 3 Study." November 9, 2020. https://www.pfizer.com/news/press-release/press-release-detail/pfizer-and-biontech-announce-vaccine-candidate-against

Pfizer. "Pfizer and BioNTech Celebrate First Authorization in the U.S. of Vaccine to Prevent COVID-19." December 11, 2020. https://www.pfizer.com/news/press-release/press-release-detail/pfizer-and-biontech-celebrate-historic-first-authorization

Pfizer, "Pfizer and BioNTech Confirm High Efficacy and No Serious Safety Concerns through up to Six Months Following Second Dose in Updated Topline Analysis of Landmark COVID-19 Vaccine Study." April 1, 2021. https://investors.pfizer.com/Investors/News/news-details/2021/Pfizer-and-BioNTech-Confirm-High-Efficacy-and-No-Serious-Safety-Concerns-Through-Up-to-Six-Months-Following-Second-Dose-in-Updated-Topline-Analysis-of-Landmark-COVID-19-Vaccine-Study-04-01-2021/default.aspx

Pfizer. "US FDA Grants Priority Review for the Biologics License Application for Pfizer BioNTech COVID-19 Vaccine." July 16, 2021. https://cdn.pfizer.com

Pfizer. "Pfizer and Biontech Announce Submission of Initial Data to US FDA to Support Booster Dose of COVID-19 Vaccine." August 16, 2021. https://www.pfizer.com/news/press-release/press-release-detail/pfizer-and-biontech-announce-submission-initial-data-us-fda

Pfizer. "Pfizer-BioNTech COVID-19 Vaccine Comirnaty™ Receives Full US FDA Approval for Individuals 16 Years and Older." August 23, 2021. https://www.pfizer.com/news/press-release/press-release-detail/pfizer-biontech-covid-19-vaccine-comirnatyr-receives-full

Pfizer. "Annual Report." 2021. https://investors.pfizer.com/Investors/Financials/Annual Reports/default.aspx

Pfizer. "Board Member: James C. Smith." 2022. https://www.pfizer.com/people/leadership/board_of_directors/james_smith

Pfizer. "Pfizer and BioNTech Initiate Rolling Submission for Emergency Use Authorization of Their COVID-19 Vaccine in Children 6 Months through 4 Years of Age Following Request from U.S. FDA." February 1, 2022. https://www.pfizer.com/news/press-release/press-release-detail/pfizer-and-biontech-initiate-rolling-submission-emergency

Pfizer. "Statement from Pfizer Chairman and CEO Albert Bourla on Testing Positive for COVID-19." August 15, 2022. https://www.pfizer.com/news/announcements/statement-pfizer-chairman-and-ceo-albert-bourla-testing-positive-covid-19

Pharmaceutical Technology. "Moderna Reports $18.5bn Total Revenue in Full-Year 2021." February 25, 2022. https://www.pharmaceutical-technology.com/news/moderna-reports-revenue-2021/

Pierson, Ransdell. "Pfizer to Settle Bextra, Celebrex Lawsuits." Reuters, October 17, 2008. https://www.reuters.com/article/us-pfizer-bextra/pfizer-to-settle-bextra-celebrex-lawsuits-idUSTRE49G43220081017

Polack, Fernando, Stephen J. Thomas, Nicholas Kitchin, Judith Absalom, Alejandra Gurtman, Stephen Lockhart, John L. Perez, et al. "Safety and Efficacy of the BNT162b2 mRNA Covid-19 Vaccine." *New England Journal of Medicine* 383, (December 31, 2020): 2603-2615. https://www.nejm.org/doi/full/10.1056/nejmoa2034577

Pollack, Andrew. "AstraZeneca Makes a Bet on an Untested Technique." *New York Times*, March 21, 2013, B7.

Reddy, Sumathi. "Over Two Million Americans Aren't Working Due to Long Covid; Brookings Institution Report Says the Loss of Work Translates into Roughly $170 Billion a Year in Lost Wages." *Wall Street Journal*, August 25,

2022. https://www.wsj.com/articles/over-2-million-americans-arent-work-ing-due-to-long-covid-says-brookings-11661364528

Regev-Yochay, Gili, Tal Gonen, Mayan Gilboa, Michal Mandelboim, Victoria Indenbaum, Sharon Amit, Lilac Meltzer, et al. "Efficacy of a Fourth Dose of Covid-19 mRNA Vaccine against Omicron." *New England Journal of Medicine* 385, no. 14 (April 7, 2022): 1377-1380. https://doi.org/10.1056/NEJMc2202542

Reidy, Chris. "Alexion, Moderna Announce Agreement to Develop Messenger RNA Therapeutics." boston.com, January 13, 2014. https://www.boston.com/news/innovation/2014/01/13/alexion-moderna-announce-agree-ment-to-develop-messenger-rna-therapeutics/

Reuter, Dominick. "Fauci Says US Is 'Perilously Close' to Doctors Having to Prioritize People for ICU Beds." *Business Insider*, September 6, 2021. https://www.businessinsider.com/fauci-says-us-doctors-may-have-to-prior-itize-icu-beds-2021-9

Reuters. "Moderna Receives $483 Million BARDA Awarded for COVID-19 Vaccine Development." April 16, 2020. https://www.reuters.com/article/us-health-coronavirus-moderna-funding/moderna-receives-483-million-barda-award-for-covid-19-vaccine-development-idUSKBN21Y3E0

Reuters. "Fact Check—Pages of Suspected Side Effects Released About Pfizer's COVID-19 Vaccine 'May Not Have Any Causal Relationship' to the Jab, Company Says." March 17, 2022. https://www.reuters.com/article/factcheck-coronavirus-pfizer/fact-check-pages-of-suspected-side-effects-released-about-pfizers-covid-19-vaccine-may-not-have-any-causal-relation-ship-to-the-jab-company-says-idUSL2N2VK1G1

Reuters. "US CDC Advisers Approve Adding Covid Shots to Vaccine Schedule." October 20, 2022. https://www.reuters.com/world/us/us-cdc-ad-visers-approve-adding-covid-shots-vaccine-schedules-2022-10-20/

Riemersma, Kasen K., Brittany E. Grogan, Amanda Kita-Yarbro, Peter J. Halfmann, Hannah E. Segaloff, Anna Kocharian, Kelsey R. Florek, et al. "Shedding of Infectious SARS-CoV-2 Despite Vaccination." medRxiv preprint, August 24, 2021. https://www.medrxiv.org/content/10.1101/2021.07.31.21261387v4

Roan, Shari. "Swine Flu 'Debacle' of 1976 Is Recalled." *Los Angeles Times*, April 27, 2009. https://www.latimes.com/archives/la-xpm-2009-apr-27-sci-swine-history27-story.html

Robbins, Rebecca, and Jenny Gross. "Moderna Sues Pfizer and BioNTech over Coronavirus Vaccine." *New York Times*, August 27, 2022, B1.

Roche, Darragh. "Members of Congress and Their Staff Are Exempt from Biden's Vaccine Mandate." *Newsweek*, September 10, 2021. https://www.newsweek.com/members-congress-staff-exempt-biden-covid-vaccine-mandate-1627859

Rosenstiel, Tom, William Buzenberg, Marjorie Connelly, and Kevin Loker. "Charting New Ground: The Ethical Terrain of Nonprofit Journalism." American Press Institute, April 20, 2016. https://www.americanpressinstitute.org/publications/reports/nonprofit-news/

Rozsa, Lori. "DeSantis Forms Panel to Counter CDC, a Move Decried by Health Professionals." *Washington Post*, December 13, 2022.

Sagonosky, Eric. "'Warp Speed' Head Slaoui, Challenged for 'Huge Conflict of Interest,' Sells off $12.4M in Moderna Stock." *Fierce Pharma*, May 19, 2020. https://www.fiercepharma.com/pharma/warp-speed-head-slaoui-divests-12-4m-moderna-holdings-to-avoid-conflict-interest

Say, Daniela, Nigel Crawford, Sarah McNab, Danielle Wurzel, Andrew Steer, and Shidan Tosif. "Post-Acute COVID-19 Outcomes in Children with Mild and Asymptomatic Disease." *Lancet: Child and Adolescent Health* 5, (June 2021): 22-23. https://doi.org/10.1016/S2352-4642(21)00124-3

Science-Based Medicine. "About SBM." Accessed June 16, 2022. https://sciencebasedmedicine.org/about-science-based-medicine/

Scientific Advisory Group for Emergencies. "Options for Increasing Adherence to Social Distancing Measures." March 22, 2020. https://www.gov.uk/government/publications/options-for-increasing-adherence-to-social-distancing-measures-22-march-2020

Scientific Advisory Group for Emergencies. "Eighty-Third SAGE Meeting on COVID-19." March 11, 2021. https://www.gov.uk/government/publications/sage-83-minutes-coronavirus-covid-19-response-11-march-2021/sage-83-minutes-coronavirus-covid-19-response-11-march-2021

Seattle Times. "Pfizer to Pay $2.3 B to Settle Fraud Case." September 3, 2009. https://www.seattletimes.com/seattle-news/health/pfizer-to-pay-23b-to-settle-fraud-case/

Segraves, Mark. "DC Offers Free Beer at Kennedy Center for Getting Vaccine." *NBC News Washington*, May 4, 2021. https://www.nbcwashington.com/news/coronavirus/dc-offers-free-beer-at-kennedy-center-for-getting-vaccine/2661082/

Sehgal, Neil Jay, Dahai Yue, Ren Hao Wang, and Dylan H. Roby. "The Association between COVID-19 Mortality and the County-Level Partisan Divide in the United States." *Health Affairs* 41, no 6 (June 2022). https://doi.org/10.1377/hlthaff.2022.00085

Shah, Anand, Peter Marks, and Stephen Hahn. "Ensuring the Safety and Effectiveness of a COVID-19 Vaccine." *Health Affairs*, August 18, 2020. https://www.healthaffairs.org/do/10.1377/forefront.20200814.996612/full/

Shaheen, Mansur. "Pfizer and Moderna Launch Trials to Track Whether Health Issues Arise YEARS after Getting Their Covid Vaccines." *Daily Mail*, November 14, 2022. https://www.dailymail.co.uk/health/article-11426007/Pfizer-Moderna-launch-trials-track-issues-arise-YEARS-getting-vaccines.html

Shimabukuro, Tom. "COVID-19 Vaccine Safety Updates." June 10, 2021. https://cdc.gov/coronavirus

Shrestha, Nabin, Patrick C. Burke, Amy S. Nowacki, James F. Simon, Amanda Hagen, and Steven M. Gordon. "Effectiveness of the Coronavirus Disease (COVID-19) Bivalent Vaccine." medRxiv preprint, December 19, 2022. https://www.medrxiv.org/content/10.1101/2022.12.17.22283625v1.full.pdf

Simonsen, Lone, Thomas A. Reichert, Cecile Viboud, William C. Blackwelder, Robert J. Taylor, and Mark A. Miller. "Impact of Influenza Vaccination on Seasonal Mortality in the US Elderly Population." *Archives of Internal Medicine* 165, no. 3 (February 14, 2005): 265-272. https://doi.org/10.1001/archinte.165.3.265

Smith, Claire, David Odd, Rachel Harwood, Joseph Ward, Michael Linney, Matthew Clark, Dougal Hargreave, et al. "Deaths in Children and Young People in England Following SARS-CoV-2 During the First Pandemic

Year: A National Study Using Linked Mandatory Child Death Reporting Data." medRxiv preprint, July 8, 2021. https://www.medrxiv.org/content/10.1101/2021.07.07.21259779v1

Smith, Hannah. "Post Claiming the Pfizer Vaccine Has Only a 12% Efficacy Rate Is Inaccurate." May 17, 2022. https://fullfact.org/health/pfizer-vaccine-efficacy/

Smith, Jennifer, and Natalie Rahhal. "FDA Panel Votes to Give Emergency Approval to Pfizer's Coronavirus Vaccine—but the Shot Won't Ship to Americans until the Agency Signs off and a Final Verdict Could Take DAYS." *Daily Mail*, December 10, 2020. https://www.dailymail.co.uk/news/article-9039119/FDA-commissioner-suggests-Pfizer-vaccine-not-approved-today.html =

Snow, John. "Cholera and the Water Supply in the South Districts of London in 1854." *Journal of Public Health and Sanitary Review* 2, no. 7 (October 1856): 239-257.

Soave, Robby. "CNN's Leana Wen: The Unvaccinated Should Not Be Allowed to Leave Their Homes." *Reason*, September 10, 2021. https://reason.com/2021/09/10/cnn-leana-wen-unvaccinated-travel-outdoor-ban/

Sorace, Stephen. "Pfizer CEO Albert Bourla Tests Positive for COVID-19 for the Second Time in Less Than Two Months." Fox Business, September 25, 2022. https://www.foxbusiness.com/business-leaders/pfizer-ceo-albert-bourla-tests-positive-covid-19-second-time-less-than-2-months

Spectator. "Hospitals Get Paid More to List Patients as COVID-19 and Three Times as Much if Patient Goes on Ventilator." April 9, 2020. https://thespectator.info/2020/04/09/hospitals-get-paid-more-to-list-patients-as-covid-19-and-three-times-as-much-if-the-patient-goes-on-ventilator-video/?utm_source=wnd&utm_medium=wnd&utm_campaign=syndicated

Speights, Keith. "Stocks the Bill & Melinda Gates Foundation Is Betting on." September 24, 2020. https://www.fool.com/investing/2020/09/24/4-coronavirus-vaccine-stocks-the-bill-melinda-gate/

Staton, Tracy. "Pfizer Settles 2,000-Plus Chantix Suits, Takes $273M Charge." *Fierce Pharma*, May 4, 2013. https://www.fiercepharma.com/sales-and-marketing/pfizer-settles-2-000-plus-chantix-suits-takes-273m-charge

Steenhuysen, Julie. "Moderna COVID-19 Vaccine Appears to Clear Safety Hurdle in Mouse Study." Reuters, June 12, 2020. https://www.reuters.com/ article/us-health-coronavirus-moderna/moderna-covid-19-vaccine-appears-to-clear-safety-hurdle-in-mouse-study-idUSKBN23J2S4

Stepleton, J.T. "Where There's Smoke, There's Big Tobacco… and Pharma and Telecom." followthemoney.org, September 9, 2017. https://www.followthemoney.org/research/blog/where-theres-smoke-theres-big-tobacco-and-pharma-and-telecom

Stieber, Zachary. "Pfizer Trial Whistleblower Presses forward with Lawsuit without Government Help." *Epoch Times*, February 14, 2022. https://www.theepochtimes.com/mkt_app/exclusive-pfizer-trial-whistleblower-presses-forward-with-lawsuit-without-us-governments-help_4277153.html

Stieber, Zachary. "Fauci, Other US Officials Served in Lawsuit over Alleged Collusion to Suppress Free Speech." *Epoch Times*, July 21, 2022. https://www.theepochtimes.com/fauci-other-us-officials-served-in-lawsuit-over-alleged-collusion-to-suppress-free-speech_4612827.html

Stieber, Zachary. "EXCLUSIVE: CDC Says It Performed Vaccine Safety Data Mining after Saying It Didn't." *Epoch Times*, July 23, 2022. https://www.theepochtimes.com/mkt_morningbrief/exclusive-cdc-says-it-performed-vaccine-safety-data-mining-after-saying-it-didnt_4617563.html

Stieber, Zachary. "EXCLUSIVE: CDC Finds Hundreds of Safety Signals for Pfizer and Moderna COVID-19 Vaccines." *Epoch Times*, January 3, 2023. https://www.theepochtimes.com/health/exclusive-cdc-finds-hundreds-of-safety-signals-for-pfizer-and-moderna-covid-19-vaccines_4956733.html

Stolberg, Sherry Gay, and Rebecca Robbins. "Moderna Moves for Total Credit in Vaccine Patent." *New York Times*, November 10, 2021.

Stone, Will. "Evidence Grows That Vaccines Lower the Risk of Getting Long Covid." National Public Radio, March 24, 2022. https://www.npr.org/sections/health-shots/2022/03/24/1088270403/long-covid-vaccines

Strong, Rebecca. "Putting Big Bad Pharma Back on Trial." Medium, February 16, 2021. https://medium.com/@bexstrong/big-pharma-corruption-and-lawsuits-amidst-covid-vaccine-c734a494b776

Subramanian, Anuradhaa, Krishnarajah Nirantharkumar, Sarah Hughes, Puja Myles, Tim Williams, Krishna M. Gokhale, Tom Taverner, et al. "Symptoms and Risk Factors for Long Covid in Non-Hospitalized Adults." *Nature Medicine* 28, (2022): 1706-1714. https://www.nature.com/articles/s41591-022-01909-wdhaa

Subramanian, S.V. and Akhil Kumar. "Increases in COVID-19 are Unrelated to Levels of Vaccination Across 68 Countries and 2947 Counties in the United States." *European Journal of Epidemiology* 36, (2021): 1237-1240. https://doi.org/10.1007/s10654-021-00808-7

Swenson, Ali. "Vaccines Didn't Cause Increase in Deaths and Life Insurance Payouts." *Associated Press*, January 10, 2022. https://apnews.com/article/fact-checking-692312045885?utm_campaign=SocialFlow&utm_medium=APFactCheck&utm_source=Twitter

Tamura, Tomokazu, Jumpei Ito, Keiya Uriu, Jiri Zahradnik, Izumi Kida, Hesham Nasser, Maya Shofa, et al. "Virological Characteristics of the SARS-CoV-2 XBB Variant Derived from Recombination of Two Omicron Subvariants." medRxiv preprint, December 19, 2022. https://www.biorxiv.org/content/10.1101/2022.12.27.521986v1

Tasker, John Paul. "Trudeau Accuses Conservative MPs of Standing with 'People Who Wave Swastikas.'" CBC News, February 17, 2022. https://www.cbc.ca/news/politics/trudeau-conservative-swastikas-1.6354970

Taylor, Nick Paul. "Genentech Lays $310 Million Wager on BioNTech's mRNA Cancer Vaccine Platform." *Fierce Biotech*, September 21, 2016. https://www.fiercebiotech.com/biotech/genentech-lays-310-million-wager-biontech-s-mrna-cancer-vaccine-platform

Thacker, Paul D. "Revelations of Poor Practices at a Contract Research Company Helping to Carry out Pfizer's Pivotal Covid-19 Vaccine Trial Raise Questions about Data Integrity and Regulatory Oversight." *BMJ* 2021;375:n2635

Thomas, Katie. "Scientists Urge Data Transparency on Vaccines to Increase Public Trust." *New York Times*, September 14, 2020, A1.

Thomas, Stephen J., Edson D. Moreira Jr., Nicholas Kitchin, Judith Absalom, Alejandra Gurtman, Stephen Lockhart, John L. Perez, et al. "Six Month

Safety and Efficacy of the BNT162b2 mRNA COVID-19 Vaccine." medRxiv preprint, July 28, 2021. https://www.medrxiv.org/content/10.1101/2021.07.28.21261159v1

Thrush, Glen. "Homelessness in US Rose for 4ᵗʰ Straight Year," *New York Times*, March 18, 2021.

Tilley, Caitlin. "Moderna's CEO Admits Only the Vulnerable Need a Covid Booster and Likens the Virus to the Flu." *Daily Mail*, October 18, 2022. https://www.dailymail.co.uk/health/article-11327615/Modernas-CEO-admits-vulnerable-need-Covid-booster-shot.html

Topley, William W.C. and Graham S. Wilson. "The Spread of Infection. The Problem of Herd Immunity." *Journal of Hygiene* 2, (1923): 243-249. https://doi.org/10.1017/S0022172400031478

Topol, Eric, and Paul Offit. "Paul Offit's Biggest Concern about Covid Vaccines." Medscape, September 9, 2020. https://www.medscape.com/viewarticle/936937

Toronto Star. "Simmering Divide over Who Isn't Vaccinated." August 26, 2021.

Trogstad, Lill. "Increased Occurrence of Menstrual Disturbances in 18- to 30-Year-Old Women after COVID-19 Vaccination." SSRN, January 14, 2022. https://papers.ssrn.com/sol3/papers.cfm?abstract_id=3998180

Tseng, Hung Fu, Bradley K. Ackerson, Katia Bruxvoort, Lina S. Sy, Julia E. Tubert, Gina S. Lee, Jennifer H. Ku, et al. "Effectiveness of mRNA-1273 against Infection and COVID-19 Hospitalization with SARS-CoC-2 Omicron Subvariants: BA.1, BA.2, BA.2.12.1, BA.4, and BA.5." medRxiv preprint, October 1, 2022. https://www.medrxiv.org/content/10.1101/2022.09.30.22280573v1.full.pdf

Tucker, Jeffrey A. "WHO Deletes Naturally Acquired Immunity from Its Website." Maine Wire, December 28, 2020. https://www.themainewire.com/2020/12/deletes-naturally-acquired-immunity-website/

Tufeki, Zeynep. "There's Terrific News about the New Covid Boosters." *New York Times*, September 16, 2022, A22.

Tulp, Sophia. "Experts Say Changes to CDC's Vaccination Definition are Normal." Associated Press, February 9, 2022. https://apnews.com/article/fact-checking-976069264061

UK Health Security Agency. "COVID-19 Vaccine Surveillance Report: Week 3." January 20, 2022.

United States Department of Defense. "US Government Engages Pfizer to Produce Millions of Doses of COVID-19 Vaccine." July 22, 2020. https://www.defense.gov/News/Releases/Release/Article/2310994/us-government-engages-pfizer-to-produce-millions-of-doses-of-covid-19-vaccine/

United States Department of Health and Human Services. "Secretarial Directive on Availability of Booster Doses of COVID-19 Vaccines." November 21, 2021. https://www.hhs.gov/sites/default/files/secretarial-directive-availability-booster-doses-covid-19-vaccines.pdf

United States Department of Health and Human Services. "Secretarial Directive on Availability of Booster Doses of COVID-19 Vaccines." December 10, 2021. https://www.hhs.gov/sites/default/files/secretarial-directive-availability-booster-doses-covid-19-vaccines-december-2021.pdf

United States Department of Health and Human Services. "Vaccine Side Effects." Page last updated May 6, 2022. https://www.hhs.gov/immunization/basics/safety/side-effects/index.html

United States Department of Health and Human Services. "Secretarial Directive on Pediatric and Second COVID-19 Vaccine Booster Doses." May 23, 2022. https://www.hhs.gov/sites/default/files/secretarial-directive-on-pediatric-and-second-booster-dose.pdf

United States Department of Health and Human Services. "Secretarial Directive on Pediatric COVID-19 Vaccines for Children 6 Months through 4/5 Years of Age." June 18, 2022.

United States Department of Justice. "Justice Department Announces Largest Health Care Fraud Settlement in Its History." September 2, 2009. https://www.justice.gov/opa/pr/justice-department-announces-largest-health-care-fraud-settlement-its-history

Valenti, Jessica. "Unvaxxed, Unmasked, and Putting Our Kids at Risk." *New York Times*, August 1, 2021.

Venkatesan, Priya. "Do Vaccines Prevent Long Covid?" *Lancet Respiratory Medicine* 10, (January 22, 2022): e30. https://doi.org/10.1016/S2213-2600(22)00020-0

Vogel, Gretchen. "Omicron Booster Shots Are Coming—with Lots of Questions." *Science*, August 30, 2022. https://www.science.org/content/article/omicron-booster-shots-are-coming-lots-questions

Wagner, Karen Dineen, Paul Ambrosini, Moira Rynn, Christopher Wohlberg, Ruoyong Yang, Michael S. Greenbaum, Ann Childress, et al. "Efficacy of Sertraline in the Treatment of Children and Adolescents with Major Depressive Disorder: Two Randomized Controlled Trials." *JAMA* 290, no. 8 (August 27, 2003): 1033-1041. https://doi.org/10.1001/jama.290.8.1033

Wall Street Journal. "How Fauci and Collins Shut Down Covid Debate: They Worked with Media to Trash the Great Barrington Declaration." December 21, 2020.

Wang, Yuxi, John Bye, Karam Bales, Deepti Gurdasani, Adityavarman Mehta, Mohammed Abba-Aji, David Stuckler, and Martin McKee. "Understanding and Neutralising Covid-19 Misinformation and Disinformation." *BMJ* 2022;379e070331

Wastila, Linda, Peter Doshi, Hamid A. Merchant, and Kim Witczak. "Why We Petitioned the FDA to Refrain from Fully Approving Any Covid-19 Vaccine This Year." *BMJ Blogs*, June 8, 2021. https://blogs.bmj.com/bmj/2021/06/08/why-we-petitioned-the-fda-to-refrain-from-fully-approving-any-covid-19-vaccine-this-year/

Wastila, Linda, Peter Doshi, Hamid A. Merchant, Kim Witczak, Anthony J. Brookes, Byram W. Bridle, Peter Collignon, et al. "Citizen Petition." June 1, 2021. https://www.regulations.gov/docket/FDA-2021-P-0521/document

Weiland, Noah. "F.D.A. Wants Covid Boosters Updated to Target Subvariants." *New York Times*, July 1, 2022, A13.

Weiland, Noah. "Biden Administration Plant to Offer New Booster Shots in September." *New York Times*, July 29, 2022, A17.

Whelan, Patrick. "Re: Notice of Meeting; Establishment of a Public Docket; Request for Comments Related to Consideration of Vaccines against

SARS-CoV-2." December 8, 2020. https://www.regulations.gov/document/FDA-2020-N-1898-0246

White House. "Press Briefing by Press Secretary Jen Psaki." July 16, 2021. https://www.whitehouse.gov/briefing-room/press-briefings/2021/07/16/press-briefing-by-press-secretary-jen-psaki-july-16-2021/

White House. "Remarks by President Biden in a CNN Town Hall with Don Lemon." July 22, 2021. https://www.whitehouse.gov/briefing-room/speeches-remarks/2021/07/22/remarks-by-president-biden-in-a-cnn-town-hall-with-don-lemon/

White House. "Press Briefing by Press Secretary Karine Jean-Pierre, COVID-19 Response Coordinator Dr. Ashish Jha, and Chief Medical Advisor Dr. Anthony Fauci." November 22, 2022. https://www.whitehouse.gov/briefing-room/press-briefings/2022/11/22/press-briefing-by-press-secretary-karine-jean-pierre-covid-19-response-coordinator-dr-ashish-jha-and-chief-medial-advisor-dr-anthony-fauci/

Wiseman, Paul. "US Jobless Claims Rise to 744k as COVID-19 Layoffs Continue." *Chicago Tribune*, April 8, 2021. https://www.chicagotribune.com/business/ct-biz-covid-unemployment-toll-20210408-n2hgwl334bhazpsapz-movwtzqm-story.htm

Witczak, Kim. "Reflections on FDA Chantix Hearing." Selling Sickness, accessed June 14, 2022. http://sellingsickness.com/reflections-on-fda-chantix-hearing/

Wolf, Naomi. *The Bodies of Others: The New Authoritarians, COVID-19, and the War against the Human.* Fort Lauderdale: All Seasons Press, May 31, 2022.

World Health Organization. "WHO Director-General's Remarks at the Media Briefing on 2019 n-CoV on 11 February 2020." February 11, 2020. https://www.who.int/director-general/speeches/detail/who-director-general-s-remarks-at-the-media-briefing-on-2019-ncov-on-11-february-2020

World Health Organization. "A Clinical Case Definition of Post COVID-19 Condition by a Delphi Consensus." October 6, 2021.

World Health Organization. "Classification of Omicron (B.1.1.529): SARS-Cov-2 Variant of Concern." November 26, 2021. https://www.who.

int/news/item/26-11-2021-classification-of-omicron-(b.1.1.529)-sars-cov-2-variant-of-concern

World Health Organization. "COVID-19 Vaccines Advice." Updated April 13, 2022. https://www.who.int/emergencies/diseases/novel-coronavirus-2019/covid-19-vaccines/advice

Wu, Fan, Su Zhao, Bin Yu, Yan-Mei Chen, Wen Wang, Zhi-Gang Song, Yi Hu, et al. "A New Coronavirus Associated with Human Respiratory Diseases in China." *Nature* 579, no. 7798 (March 12, 2020): 265-269. https://doi.org/10.1038/s41586-020-2008-3

Wu, Katherine J. "The Worst Pediatric-Care Crisis in Decades." *Atlantic*, October 31, 2022.

Wu, Zhunyou, and Jennifer McGoogan. "Characteristics of and Important Lessons from the Coronavirus Disease 2019 (COVID-19) Outbreak in China: Summary of a Report of 72,314 Cases from the Chinese Center for Disease Control and Prevention." *JAMA* 323, no. 13 (February 24, 2020): 1239-1242. https://doi.org/10.1001/jama.2020.2648

Yahoo Finance. "BioNTech SE (BNTX)." Accessed May 28, 2022. https://finance.yahoo.com/quote/BNTX/key-statistics/

Younes, Jenin. "The U.S. Government's Vast New Privatized Censorship Regime." *Tablet*, September 21, 2022. https://www.tabletmag.com/sections/arts-letters/articles/government-privatized-censorship-regime

YouTube. July 22, 2022. https://www.youtube.com/shorts/x8Sl9DORB_

Ziady, Hanna. "Covid Vaccine Profits Mint 9 New Pharma Billionaires." Reuters, May 21, 2021. https://www.cnn.com/2021/05/21/business/covid-vaccine-billionaires/index.html

Zuckerman, Gregory. *A Shot to Save the World: The Inside Story of the Life-or-Death Race for a Covid-19 Vaccine.* New York: Penguin Random House, October 26, 2021.

Index

E

Epoch Times, 139, 166, 167, 184, 240, 284, 327, 331, 338

F

Facebook, 74, 92, 105, 159, 176, 182

Fauci, Anthony, 17, 18, 67, 83, 90, 115-118, 132, 153, 156, 166, 169, 188, 233-235, 243, 275, 280, 284, 288, 289, 318, 323, 331, 337

Flagship Pioneering (Flagship Ventures), 53, 54, 74

Food and Drug Administration (FDA), ii, 6-9, 15-16, 20, 24, 38, 41-53, 62-65, 69, 72-79, 84-94, 99-104, 109, 113, 127-132, 136-142, 148, 153, 157, 161, 164-165, 169, 172-174, 181-186, 189, 196-200, 203, 216-222, 225, 236, 242-246, 252-255, 259, 260-270, 278-279, 283, 288-289, 303-309, 314-320, 326, 327, 331-332

G

Gates, Bill, 31, 259-298, 305

Gorski, David, 22-23, 117, 157-158, 225, 264, 304, 323, 330, 336

Gottlieb, Scott, 45, 132, 242-243, 253, 338

Great Barrington Declaration, 117, 166, 169, 189, 234, 239, 240, 270, 288, 323

Gupta, Sunetra, 117, 189, 270, 323

H

Hahn, Stephen, 6, 24, 74, 77, 236, 268-270, 282, 301, 305, 315, 340

Harper, Phil, 46, 160, 162, 254, 265, 329, 330

Health Advisory and Recovery Team (HART) Group, 143, 265, 328-329

Healy, David, 8-9, 21, 42, 69, 79, 90, 98, 103, 109, 128, 130, 140-146, 195, 220, 247, 259, 265-268, 301, 304, 322, 326-328, 337-339

Herd Immunity, 273, 286, 304

Høeg v Newsom, 229, 231, 252

I

Ischemic stroke, 240

J

K

L

M

Rubin, Eric, 88

S

Schwarzenegger, Arnold, 76, 251, 316

Scientific Advisory Group for Emergencies (SAGE), 4, 59, 281, 312

Snow, John, 117, 251, 283, 323

Spike protein, 5, 27, 29-39, 62-64, 68-71, 77, 89, 91, 106, 119, 136, 138, 143, 162, 172, 185, 197, 208, 241, 245-246

T

T-cells, 58, 197

Thomson Reuters Foundation, 77

Topol, Eric, 10, 44, 286, 301

Toronto Star, 76, 82, 125, 271, 277, 286, 316-317, 326

Trudeau, Justin, 110, 141-142, 262, 276, 285, 322, 328

Tucker, Jeffrey, 19, 203, 286, 304

Twitter, 68, 82, 103, 107, 160-162, 177, 182, 185-188, 229-234, 239, 240, 242, 243, 253, 285, 325, 338

V

Vaccine Adverse Event Reporting System (VAERS), 34-36, 65, 70-73, 89, 110, 138-140, 146, 153-159, 165-167, 245, 246

Ventavia Research Group, 101-103, 139, 200-203, 231

W

Walensky, Rochelle, 61, 132, 153, 165-167, 184, 226, 276, 336

Wastila, Linda, iii, 69, 72, 80, 90-92, 195-200, 288, 314, 339

Witczak, Kim, ii, 16, 52, 69, 72, 78, 90, 99, 217, 288-289, 309

Wolf, Naomi, 193, 289, 336

Woodcock, Janet, 24, 78, 132, 268, 305

World Health Organization (WHO), 19, 116, 274, 286, 289, 299, 304

Wuhan, 1, 2, 164, 172-173, 259, 267, 298

296

Y

Z

Endnotes

1   Chaolin Huang et al., "Clinical Features of Patients Infected with 2019 Novel Coronavirus in Wuhan, China," *Lancet* 395, no. 10223 (February 15, 2020): 497-506, https://doi.org/10.1016/S0140-6736(20)30183-5

2   Zunyou Wu and Jennifer McGoogan, "Characteristics of and Important Lessons from the Coronavirus Disease 2019 (COVID-19) Outbreak in China: Summary of a Report of 72,314 Cases from the Chinese Center for Disease Control and Prevention," *JAMA* 323, no. 13 (February 24, 2020): 1239-1242, https://doi.org/10.1001/jama.2020.2648

3   Fan Wu et al., "A New Coronavirus Associated with Human Respiratory Diseases in China," *Nature* 579, no. 7798 (March 12, 2020): 265-269, https://doi.org/10.1038/s41586-020-2008-3

4   Bo Li et al., "Prevalence and Impact of Cardiovascular Metabolic Diseases on COVID-19 in China," *Clinical Research in Cardiology* 109, no. 5 (May 2020): 531-538, https://doi.org/10.1007/s00392-020-01626-9

5   Coalition for Epidemic Preparedness Innovations, "CEPI to Fund Three Programmes to Develop Three Vaccines against the Novel Coronavirus, nCoV-2019," January 23, 2020, https://cepi.net/news_cepi/cepi-to-fund-three-programmes-to-develop-vaccines-against-the-novel-coronavirus-ncov-2019/

6   Andrew Dunn, "A Coalition Backed by Bill Gates Is Funding Biotechs That Are Scrambling to Develop Vaccines for the Deadly Wuhan Cornonavirus," *Business Insider India*, January 23, 2020, https://www.businessinsider.in/science/news/a_coalition_backed_by_bill_gates_is_

funding_biotechs_that_are_scrambling_to_develop_vaccines_for_the_
deadly_wuhan_cornonavirus/articleshow/73559156.cms

7   Coronavirus Study Group, "Severe Acute Respiratory Syndrome-Related Coronavirus: The Species and Its Viruses," February 11, 2020, https://www.biorxiv.org/content/10.1101/2020.02.07.937862v1

8   World Health Organization, "WHO Director-General's Remarks at the Media Briefing on 2019-n-CoV on 11 February 2020," February 11, 2020, https://www.who.int/director-general/speeches/detail/who-direc-tor-general-s-remarks-at-the-media-briefing-on-2019-ncov-on-11-feb-ruary-2020

9   Alex Berenson, *Pandemia: How Coronavirus Hysteria Took over Our Government, Rights, and Lives* (Washington DC: Regnery Publishing, November 30, 2021).

10   Paul Wiseman, "US Jobless Claims Rise to 744k as COVID-19 Layoffs Continue," *Chicago Tribune*, April 8, 2021, https://www.chicagotribune.com/business/ct-biz-covid-unemployment-toll-20210408-n2hgwl-334bhazpsapzmovwtzqm-story.html; Glen Thrush, "Homelessness in US Rose for 4th Straight Year," *New York Times*, March 18, 2021; Sasha Pezenik, "Alcohol Consumption Rising Sharply during Pandemic, Especially among Women," ABC News, September 29, 2020, https://abcnews.go.com/US/alcohol-consumption-rising-sharply-pandem-ic-women/story?id=73302479; Mark É. Czeisler et al., "Mental Health, Substance Abuse, and Suicidal Ideation during the COVID-19 Pandemic – United States, June 24-30, 2020," *Morbidity and Mortality Weekly Report* 69, no. 32 (1049-1057), https://www.cdc.gov/mmwr/volumes/69/wr/mm6932a1.htm; Express Scripts, "America's State of Mind: US Trends in Medication Use for Depression, Anxiety, and Insomnia," April 2020, https://corporate-site-labs-prod.s3.us cast 2.amazonaws.com/2020-04/Express%20Scripts%20America%27s%20State%20of%20Mind%20Report%20April%202020%20FINAL_1.pdf

11   Scientific Advisory Group for Emergencies, "Options for Increasing Adherence to Social Distancing Measures," March 22, 2020, https://www.gov.uk/government/publications/options-for-increasing-adherence-to-so-cial-distancing-measures-22-march-2020

12   Anna Merlan, "Anti-Vaxxers Are Terrified the Government Will Enforce a Vaccine for Coronavirus," *Vice*, February 28, 2020, https://www.vice.com/en/article/m7q5vv/anti-vaxxers-are-terrified-the-government-will-enforce-a-vaccine-for-coronavirus

13   Derek Cheng, "Coronavirus: Jacinda Ardern Dismisses Nationwide Lockdown Speculation on Social Media," *New Zealand Herald*, March 18, 2020, https://www.nzherald.co.nz/nz/coronavirus-jacinda-ardern-dismisses-nationwide-lockdown-speculation-on-social-media/I2FTKPSA36LJIDNLBFIYECXDHM/

14   *New Zealand Herald*, "New Zealand Enters Nationwide Lockdown in Fight against COVID-19," March 25, 2020, https://nzhistory.govt.nz/page/new-zealand-enters-nationwide-lockdown-fight-against-covid-19

15   National Institute of Allergies and Infectious Disease, "NIH Clinical Trial of Investigational Vaccine for COVID-19 Begins," March 16, 2020, https://www.niaid.nih.gov/diseases-conditions/coronaviruses

16   Denise Grady, "Testing on Humans Begins for an Experimental Vaccine," *New York Times*, March 17, 2020, A12.

17   Reuters, "Moderna Receives $483 Million BARDA Awarded for COVID-19 Vaccine Development," April 16, 2020, https://www.reuters.com/article/us-health-coronavirus-moderna-funding/moderna-receives-483-million-barda-award-for-covid-19-vaccine-development-idUSKBN21Y3E0

18   *New York Times*, "Around the World," May 7, 2020, A12.

19   Eric Sagonosky, "'Warp Speed' Head Slaoui, Challenged for 'Huge Conflict of Interest,' Sells off $12.4M in Moderna Stock," *Fierce Pharma*, May 19, 2020, https://www.fiercepharma.com/pharma/warp-speed-head-slaoui-divests-12-4m-moderna-holdings-to-avoid-conflict-interest

20   Ibid.

21   Julie Steenhuysen, "Moderna COVID-19 Vaccine Appears to Clear Safety Hurdle in Mouse Study," Reuters, June 12, 2020, https://www.reuters.com/article/us-health-coronavirus-moderna/moderna-covid-19-vaccine-appears-to-clear-safety-hurdle-in-mouse-study-idUSKBN23J2S4

22   United States Department of Defense, "US Government Engages Pfizer to Produce Millions of Doses of COVID-19 Vaccine," July 22, 2020, https://www.defense.gov/News/Releases/Release/Article/2310994/us-government-engages-pfizer-to-produce-millions-of-doses-of-covid-19-vaccine/

23   Anand Shah, Peter Marks, and Stephen Hahn, "Ensuring the Safety and Effectiveness of a COVID-19 Vaccine," *Health Affairs*, August 18, 2020, https://www.healthaffairs.org/do/10.1377/forefront.20200814.996612/full/

24   Raymond M. Johnson, Peter Doshi, and David Healy, "Covid-19: Should Doctors Recommend Treatments and Vaccines When Full Data Are Not Publicly Available?" *BMJ* 2020;370:m3260

25   David Healy, *Pharmageddon* (Berkely: University of California Press, March 12, 2012).

26   Peter Doshi et al., "Restoring Invisible and Abandoned Trials: A Call for People to Publish the Findings," *BMJ* 2013;346:f2865

27   David Healy, Joann LeNoury, and Julie Wood, *Children of the Cure: Missing Data, Lost Lives, and Antidepressants* (Toronto: Samizdat Health Writer's Co-operative, 2020).

28   Johnson et al., "Vaccines."

29   BioNTech, "Biopharma Leaders Unite to Stand with Science," September 8, 2020, https://www.globenewswire.com/news-release/2020/09/08/2089875/0/en/Biopharma-Leaders-Unite-to-Stand-with-Science.html

30   Eric Topol and Paul Offit, "Paul Offit's Biggest Concern about COVID Vaccines," Medscape, September 9, 2020, https://www.medscape.com/viewarticle/936937

31   Katie Thomas, "Scientists Urge Data Transparency on Vaccines to Increase Public Trust," *New York Times*, September 14, 2020, A1.

32   Denise Grady and Katie Thomas, "2 Firms Share Plans on Trials for a Vaccine," *New York Times*, September 18, 2020, A1.

33   Ibid.

34   Peter Doshi, "Will Covid-19 Vaccines Save Lives? Current Trials Aren't Designed to Tell Us," *BMJ* 2020;371:m4037

35   Ibid.

36   Ibid.

37   Ibid.

38   Lone Simonsen et al., "Impact of Influenza Vaccination on Seasonal Mortality in the US Elderly Population," *Archives of Internal Medicine* 165, no. 3 (February 14, 2005): 265-272, https://doi.org/10.1001/archinte.165.3.265

39   Pfizer, "Pfizer and BioNTech Announce Vaccine Candidate against COVID-19 Achieved Success in First Interim Analysis from Phase 3 Study," November 9, 2020, https://www.pfizer.com/news/press-release/press-release-detail/pfizer-and-biontech-announce-vaccine-candidate-against

40   *Axios*, "Pfizer CEO Says He Would Have Released Vaccine Data before Election if Possible," November 9, 2020, https://www.axios.com/2020/11/09/pfizer-ceo-says-he-wouldve-released-vaccine-data-before-election-if-possible

41   Moderna, "Moderna's COVID-19 Vaccine Candidate Meets Its Primary Efficacy Endpoint in the First Interim Analysis of the Phase 3 COVE Study," November 16, 2020, https://www.biospace.com/article/releases/moderna-s-covid-19-vaccine-candidate-meets-its-primary-aefficacy-endpoint-in-the-first-interim-analysis-of-the-phase-3-cove-study/

42   David Cyranoski, "Why Emergency COVID-Vaccine Approvals Pose a Dilemma for Scientists," *Nature*, November 23, 2020, https://www.nature.com/articles/d41586-020-03219-y

43   Peter Doshi, "Pfizer and Moderna's '95% Effective' Vaccines – Let's Be Cautious and First See the Full Data," *BMJ Blogs*, November 26, 2020, https://blogs.bmj.com/bmj/2020/11/26/peter-doshi-pfizer-and-modernas-95-effective-vaccines-lets-be-cautious-and-first-see-the-full-data/

44   Pfizer, "A Phase 1/2/3 Placebo-Controlled, Randomized, Observer-Blind Dose-Finding Study to Evaluate the Safety, Tolerability, Immunoge-

nicity, and Efficacy of SARS-2-CoV RNA Vaccine Candidates against COVID-19 in Healthy Individuals," accessed June 15, 2022, https://cdn. pfizer.com/pfizercom/2020-11/C4591001_Clinical_Protocol_Nov2020. pdf

45   Moderna, "A Phase 3, Randomized, Stratified, Observer-Blind, Placebo-Controlled Study to Evaluate the Efficacy, Safety, and Immunogenicity of mRNA-1273 SARS-CoV-2 Vaccine in Adults Aged 18 Years and Older," August 20, 2020, https://covid19crc.org/publications-and-resources/covid-19-studies/moderna/

46   Doshi, "95% Effective."

47   FDA, "FDA Takes Key Action in Fight against COVID-19 by Issuing Emergency Use Authorization for the First COVID-19 Vaccine," December 11, 2020, https://www.fda.gov/news-events/press-announcements/fda-takes-key-action-fight-against-covid-19-issuing-emergency-use-authorization-first-covid-19

48   Pfizer, "Pfizer and BioNTech Celebrate First Authorization in the U.S. of Vaccine to Prevent COVID-19," December 11, 2020, https://www.pfizer. com/news/press-release/press-release-detail/pfizer-and-biontech-celebrate-historic-first-authorization

49   Jennifer Smith and Natalie Rahhal, "FDA Panel Votes to Give Emergency Approval to Pfizer's Coronavirus Vaccine – but the Shot Won't Ship to Americans until the Agency Signs off and a Final Verdict Could Take DAYS," *Daily Mail,* December 10, 2020, https://www. dailymail.co.uk/news/article-9039119/FDA-commissioner-suggests-Pfizer-vaccine-not-approved-today.html

50   European Medicines Agency, "EMA Recommends First COVID-19 Vaccine for Authorisation in the EU," December 12, 2022, https://www. ema.europa.eu/en/news/ema-recommends-first-covid-19-vaccine-authorisation-eu

51   Lucy Hooker and Daniele Palumbo, "Covid Vaccines: Will Drug Companies Make Bumper Profits?" BBC Business, December 18, 2020, https:// www.bbc.com/news/business-55170756

52   Donald G. McNeil, "How Much Herd Immunity Is Enough?" *New York Times*, December 24, 2020.

53   Kansas State Agricultural College Experimental Station, "Contagious Abortion of Cattle," August 1918.

54   William W.C. Topley and Graham S. Wilson, "The Spread of Infection. The Problem of Herd Immunity," *Journal of Hygiene* 2, (1923): 243-249, https://doi.org/10.1017/S0022172400031478

55   Sheldon F. Dudley, "The Control of Diphtheria in Crowded Institutions," *Public Health* 42, (November 1928): 48-54.

56   Sheldon F. Dudley, "The Ecological Outlook on Epidemiology," *Proceedings of the Royal Society of Medicine* 30, no. 1 (1936): 57-70.

57   Jeffrey A. Tucker, "WHO Deletes Naturally Acquired Immunity from Its Website," Maine Wire, December 28, 2020, https://www.themainewire.com/2020/12/deletes-naturally-acquired-immunity-website/

58   Fernando P. Polack, et al., "Safety and Efficacy of the BNT162b2 mRNA Covid-19 Vaccine," *New England Journal of Medicine* 383, (December 31, 2020): 2603-2615, https://www.nejm.org/doi/full/10.1056/nejmoa2034577

59   Rebecca Strong, "Putting Big Bad Pharma Back on Trial," Medium, February 16, 2021, https://medium.com/@bexstrong/big-pharma-corruption-and-lawsuits-amidst-covid-vaccine-c734a494b776

60   Peter Doshi, "Pfizer and Moderna's '95% Effective Vaccines – We Need More Details and the Raw Data," *BMJ Blogs*, January 4, 2021, https://blogs.bmj.com/bmj/2021/01/04/peter-doshi-pfizer-and-modernas-95-effective-vaccines-we-need-more-details-and-the-raw-data/

61   Tucker, "Immunity."

62   David Healy, "Report Covid Vaccine Effects to RxISK," RxISK, January 11, 2021, https://rxisk.org/report-covid-vaccine-effects-to-rxisk/

63   David Gorski, "Why Is Peter Doshi Still an Editor at the BMJ?" Respectful Insolence, January 15, 2021, https://respectfulinsolence.com/2021/01/15/why-is-peter-doshi-still-an-editor-at-the-bmj/

64   See Chapter Three.

65   Science-Based Medicine, "About SBM," accessed June 16, 2022, https://
sciencebasedmedicine.org/about-science-based-medicine/

66   Jastra Kranjec, "Pfizer-BioNTech and Moderna to Earn $14.7 B in
COVID-19 Vaccine Sales by 2023," January 19, 2021, https://www.
finaria.it/pr/pfizer-biontech-and-moderna-to-earn-14-7b-from-covid-
19-vaccines-sales-by-2023/

67   Shelia Kaplan, "Hahn Leaves FDA; Woodcock Named Acting Commissioner," *New York Times*, January 20, 2021.

68   Jennifer Block, "Vaccinating People Who Have Had Covid-19: Why
Doesn't Natural Immunity Count?" *BMJ* 2021;374n:n2101

69   Edward Jenner, *An Inquiry into the Causes and Effects of the Variole Vaccinae,
or Cow-Pox* (London: Sampson and Low, 1798).

70   Derrick Baxby, "Edward Jenner's Inquiry after 200 Years," *BMJ* 318, no.
7180 (February 6, 1999): 390, https://doi.org/10.1136/bmj.318.7180.390

71   Louis Pasteur, "Sur les Maladies Virulentes et en Particulier sur la
Maladie Apellée Vulgairment Choléra des Poules," *Comptes Rendus
Hebdomaires des Séances de l'Academie des Sciences* 90, (1880): 239-248.

72   Robert Malone et al., "Cationic Liposome-Mediated RNA Transfection,"
Proceedings of the National Academy of Sciences 86, no. 16 (August 1989):
6077-6081, https://doi.org/10.1073/pnas.86/16/6077

73   Bill Gates, "Here Are the Innovations We Need to Reopen the Economy,"
Washington Post, April 23, 2020, https://www.washingtonpost.com/
opinions/2020/04/23/bill-gates-here-are-innovations-we-need-reopen-
economy/

74   Moderna, "mRNA Platform: Enabling Drug Discovery and Development," accessed April 3, 2022, https://www.modernatx.com

75   Darja Kanduc and Yehuda Schoenfeld, "Molecular Mimicry between
SARS-CoV-2 Spike Glycoprotein and Mammalian Proteomes: Implications for the Vaccine," *Immunologic Research* 68, no. 5 (2020): 310-313,
https://doi.org/1007/s12026-020-09152-6

76   Darja Kanduc, "Peptide Cross-Reactivity: The Original Sin of Vaccines," *Frontiers in Bioscience* S4, (June 1, 2021): 1393-1401, https://doi.org/10.2741/s341

77   Nikolai Eroshenko et al., "Implications of Antibody-Dependent Enhancement of Infection for SARS-CoV-2 Countermeasures," *Nature Biotechnology* 38, (July 2020): 788-797, https://doi.org/10.1038/s41587-020-0577-1

78   Ann M. Arvin et al., "A Perspective on Potential Antibody-Dependent Enhancement of SARS-CoV-2," *Nature* 584, no. 7821 (August 20, 2020): 353-363, https://doi.org/10.1038/s41586-020-2538-8

79   Patrick Whelan, "Re: Notice of Meeting; Establishment of a Public Docket; Request for Comments Related to Consideration of Vaccines against SARS-CoV-2," December 8, 2020, https://www.regulations.gov/document/FDA-2020-N-1898-024c

80   Eric L. Brown and Heather T. Essigmann, "Original Antigenic Sin: The Downside of Immunological Memory and Implications for COVID-19," *mSphere* 6, no. 2 (March 10, 2021): 1-6, https://doi.org/10/1128/mSphere.00056-21

81   SARS-CoV-2 and the RAAS. Nour Chams, Sana Chams, Reina Badran, Ali Shams, Abdallah Araji, Mohamad Raad, Sanjay Mukhopadhyay, Edana Stroberg, Eric J. Duval, Lisa M. Barton, and Inaya Hajj Hussein, CC BY 4.0 <https://creativecommons.org/licenses/by/4.0>, via Wikimedia Commons

82   FDA, "Psychopharmacological Drugs Advisory Committee: Thirty-Third Meeting," 9:00 AM Monday, November 19, 1990.

83   Karen Dineen Wagner et al., "Efficacy of Sertraline in the Treatment of Children and Adolescents with Major Depressive Disorder: Two Randomized Controlled Trials," *JAMA* 290, no. 8 (August 27, 2003): 1033-1041, https://doi.org/10.1001/jama.290.8.1033

84   United States Department of Justice, "Justice Department Announces Largest Health Care Fraud Settlement in Its History," September 2, 2009, https://www.justice.gov/opa/pr/justice-department-announces-largest-health-care-fraud-settlement-its-history

85   Matthew Herper, "Bextra! Bextra! Pharmacia Drug Approved!" *Forbes*, November 19, 2001, https://www.forbes.com/2001/11/19/1119bextra. html?sh=13d6b04f11ee

86   Melody Petersen, *Our Daily Meds* (New York: Sarah Crichton Books, 2008), 198-199.

87   Ibid., 199-201.

88   Scott Hensley, "Pfizer Makes Aid Pledge, Breaks Aid Pact," *Wall Street Journal*, November 12, 2003, B1.

89   Ibid.

90   Ibid.

91   Harris Gardiner, "Pfizer to Pay $2.3 Billion to Settle Inquiry over Marketing," *New York Times*, September 3, 2009, B4.

92   Jim Edwards, "Blue Cross Names and Shames Pfizer Execs Linked to Massages-for-Prescriptions Push," CBS News, June 10, 2010, https:// www.cbsnews.com/news/blue-cross-names-and-shames-pfizer-execs-linked-to-massages-for-prescriptions-push/

93   Alex Berenson, "Pfizer Loses One Remedy for Its Slump," *New York Times*, April 7, 2005, C1.

94   Ransdell Pierson, "Pfizer to Settle Bextra, Celebrex Lawsuits," Reuters, October 17, 2008, https://www.reuters.com/article/us-pfizer-bextra/ pfizer-to-settle-bextra-celebrex-lawsuits-idUSTRE49G43220081017

95   United States Department of Justice, "Settlement."

96   *Seattle Times*, "Pfizer to Pay $2.3 B to Settle Fraud Case," September 3, 2009, https://www.seattletimes.com/seattle-news/health/pfizer-to-pay-23b-to-settle-fraud-case/

97   Drew Griffin and Andy Segal, "Feds Found Pfizer Too Big to Nail," CNN, April 2, 2010, http://www.cnn.com/2010/HEALTH/04/02/ pfizer.bextra/index.html

98   Gardiner, "Inquiry."

99   *Seattle Times*, "Fraud."

100   Griffin and Segal, "Feds."

101   Ibid.

102   Ibid.

103   Ibid.

104   John R. MacArthur, "The Publisher's Role: Crusading Defender of the First Amendment or Advertising Salesman?" in *The Art of Making Magazines: On Being an Editor and Other Views from the Industry*, ed. Victor S. Navasky and Evan Cornog (New York: Columbia University Press, 2012), 141-153.

105   ABC News, "Girlfriend Believes Chantix Contributed to Texas Musician's Death," September 19, 2007, https://abcnews.go.com/GMA/OnCall/story?id=3623085&page=1

106   Megan Miller, "Lawsuit Claims Economy Murder-Suicide Caused by Stop-Smoking Drug," *Star-Courier*, May 9, 2011, https://www.starcourier.com/story/news/crime/2011/05/10/lawsuit-claims-economy-murder-suicide/18379085007/

107   Daily Mail, "Father Who Murdered His Family Had Been on Anti-Smoking Medication That Caused Depression," April 6, 2011, https://www.dailymail.co.uk/news/article-1373983/Father-murdered-family-quitting-smoking-medication-caused-depression.html

108   Associated Press, "Chantix, Smoking Cessation Drug, Blamed in Murder-Suicide," *Oregonian*, December 1, 2013, https://www.oregonlive.com/pacific-northwest-news/2013/11/chantix_smoking_cessation_drug.html

109   Matthew Herper, "Can Chantix Make a Comeback?" *Forbes*, September 12, 2008, https://www.forbes.com/2008/09/11/pfizer-smoking-chantix-biz-healthcare-cx_mh_0911chantix.html?sh=2f3d36be6d95

110   CBS News, "2nd Quit-Smoking Drug Gets FDA's OK," May 11, 2006, https://www.cbsnews.com/news/2nd-quit-smoking-drug-gets-fdas-ok/

111   Thomas J. Moore et al., "Strong Safety Signal Seen for Chantix (Varenicline)," *QuarterWatch*, May 25, 2008, 1-14.

112   Associated Press, "FDA Investigates Quit-Smoking Drug," *New York Times*, November 21, 2007.

113 Harris Gardiner and Duff Wilson, "FDA Warns of Side Effects for 2 Stop-Smoking Drugs," *New York Times*, July 2, 2009, B2.

114 Thomas J. Moore et al., "Thoughts and Acts of Aggression/Violence toward Others Reported in Association with Varenicline," *Annals of Pharmacotherapy* 44, no. 9 (September 2010): 1389-1394, https://doi.org/10.1345/aph.1OP172

115 Thomas J. Moore et al., "Prescription Drugs Associated with Reports of Violence towards Others," *PLoS One* 5, no. 12 (December 15, 2010), https://doi.org/10.1371/journal.pone.0015337

116 Thomas J. Moore et al., "New Varenicline (CHANTIX) Suicide Cases," *QuarterWatch*, May 19, 2011, 2.

117 Tracy Staton, "Pfizer Settles 2,000-Plus Chantix Suits, Takes $273M Charge," *Fierce Pharma*, May 4, 2013, https://www.fiercepharma.com/sales-and-marketing/pfizer-settles-2-000-plus-chantix-suits-takes-273m-charge

118 Thomas J. Moore et al., "Varenicline (CHANTIX) and Suicidal/Homicidal Thoughts," *QuarterWatch*, September 24, 2014, 2.

119 Kim Witczak, "Reflections on Fda Chantix Hearing," Selling Sickness, accessed June 14, 2022, http://sellingsickness.com/reflections-on-fda-chantix-hearing/

120 Megan Brooks, "Keep Chantix Black Box Warning, FDA Panel Says," Medscape, October 17, 2014, https://www.medscape.com/viewarticle/833402

121 FDA, "FDA Drug Safety Communication: FDA Updates Label for Stop Smoking Drug Chantix (Varenicline) to Include Potential Alcohol Interaction, Rare Risk of Seizures, and Studies of Side Effects on Mood, Behavior, or Thinking," March 9, 2015, https://www.fda.gov/drugs/drug-safety-and-availability/fda-drug-safety-communication-fda-updates-label-stop-smoking-drug-chantix-varenicline-include

122 FDA, "FDA Drug Safety Communication: FDA Revises Description of Mental Health Side Effects of the Stop-Smoking Medicines Chantix (Varenicline) and Zyban (Bupropion) to Reflect Clinical Trial Findings," December 16, 2016, https://www.fda.gov/drugs/drug-safety-and-avail-

ability/fda-drug-safety-communication-fda-revises-description-mental-health-side-effects-stop-smoking

123   Pfizer, "Annual Report," 2021, https://investors.pfizer.com/Investors/Financials/Annual-Reports/default.aspx

124   Gregory Zuckerman, *A Shot to Save the World: The Inside Story of the Life-or-Death Race for a Covid-19 Vaccine* (New York: Penguin Random House, October 26, 2021).

125   Andrew Pollack, "AstraZeneca Makes a Bet on an Untested Technique," *New York Times*, March 21, 2013, B7.

126   Damian Garde, "Ego, Ambition, and Turmoil: Inside One of Biotech's Most Secretive Startups," *STAT*, September 13, 2016, https://www.statnews.com/2016/09/13/moderna-therapeutics-biotech-mrna/

127   Chris Reidy, "Alexion, Moderna Announce Agreement to Develop Messenger RNA Therapeutics," boston.com, January 13, 2014, https://www.boston.com/news/innovation/2014/01/13/alexion-moderna-announce-agreement-to-develop-messenger-rna-therapeutics/

128   Damian Garde, "Lavishly Funded Moderna Hits Safety Problems in Bold Bid to Revolutionize Medicine," *STAT*, January 10, 2017, https://www.statnews.com/2017/01/10/moderna-trouble-mrna/

129   Ibid.

130   Ben Adams, "A Tale of 2 (Bio) Cities: Moderna Tops $100B Valuation, Matching GlaxoSmithKline," *Fierce Biotech*, July 15, 2021, https://www.fiercebiotech.com/biotech/a-tale-two-bio-cities-moderna-tops-100b-valuation-matching-glaxosmithkline

131   Pharmaceutical Technology, "Moderna Reports $18.5bn Total Revenue in Full-Year 2021," February 25, 2022, https://www.pharmaceutical-technology.com/news/moderna-reports-revenue-2021/

132   Moderna, "Moderna Reports First Quarter 2022 Financial Results and Provides Business Updates," May 4, 2022, https://investors.modernatx.com/news/news-details/2022/Moderna-Reports-First-Quarter-2022-Financial-Results-and-Provides-Business-Updates/default.aspx

133 Damian Garde, "Sanofi Inks a $1.5B Deal to Join BioNTech's Growing List of Oncology Partners," *Fierce Biotech*, November 3, 2015, https://www.fiercebiotech.com/partnering/sanofi-inks-a-1-5b-deal-to-join-bion-tech-s-growing-list-of-oncology-partners

134 Nick Paul Taylor, "Genentech Lays $310 Million Wager on BioNTech's mRNA Cancer Vaccine Platform," *Fierce Biotech*, September 21, 2016, https://www.fiercebiotech.com/biotech/genentech-lays-310-million-wager-biontech-s-mrna-cancer-vaccine-platform

135 BioNTech, "BioNTech Signs Collaborative Agreement with Pfizer to Develop mRNA-Based Vaccines for Prevention of Influenza," August 16, 2018, https://biontechse.gcs-web.com/news-releases/news-release-details/biontech-signs-collaboration-agreement-pfizer-develop-mrna-based

136 BioNTech, "BioNTech Announces Fourth Quarter and Full Year 2021 Financial Results and Corporate Update," March 30, 2022, https://investors.biontech.de/news-releases/news-release-details/biontech-announces-fourth-quarter-and-full-year-2021-financial

137 Yahoo Finance, "BioNTech SE (BNTX)," accessed May 28, 2022, https://finance.yahoo.com/quote/BNTX/key-statistics/

138 BioNTech, "Pipeline," downloaded May 28, 2022, https://www.biontech.com/content/dam/corporate/pdf/20220330_BiontechPipeline.pdf

139 Paul R. Hunter and Julii Brainard, "Estimating the Effectiveness of the Pfizer COVID-19 BNT162b2 Vaccine after a Single Dose. A Reanalysis of a Study of 'Real-World' Vaccination Outcomes from Israel," medRxiv preprint, February 3, 2021, https://www.medrxiv.org/content/10.1101/2021.02.01.21250957v1

140 Edel Kenealy, "Scots Care Home Residents Test Positive for Covid-19 Days after Receiving Vaccine," *Daily Record*, January 6, 2021, https://www.dailyrecord.co.uk/news/local-news/care-home-residents-test-positive-23269764; Ryan Evans, "Coronavirus Outbreak: 22 Deaths at Pemberley House Care Home," *Gazette*, January 27, 2021, https://www.basingstokegazette.co.uk/news/19043790.coronavirus-outbreak-22-deaths-pemberley-house-care-home/; Lisa Letcher, "Eleven Residents Die in Three Weeks after Care Home Covid Outbreak," CornwallLive,

February 15, 2021, https://www.cornwalllive.com/news/cornwall-news/eleven-residents-die-three-weeks-5005443

141   Mark J. Mulligan et al., "Phase I/II Study of COVID-19 RNA Vaccine BNT162b1 in Adults," *Nature* 586, (October 22, 2020): 589-593, https://doi.org/10.1038/s41586-020-2639-4

142   Michael Day, "Covid-19: Stronger Warnings are Needed to Curb Socializing after Vaccination, Say Doctors and Behavioural Scientists," *BMJ* 2021;372:n783

143   Jamie Lopez Bernal et al., "Early Effectiveness of COVID-19 Vaccination with BNT162b mRNA Vaccine and ChAdOx1 Adenovirus Vector Vaccine on Symptomatic Disease, Hospitalizations, and Mortality in Older Adults in England," medRxiv preprint, March 2, 2021, https://www.medrxiv.org/content/10.1101/2021.03.01.21252652v1

144   Ida Rask Moustsen-Helms et al., "Vaccine Effectiveness after 1st and 2nd Dose of the BNT162b2 mRNA COVID-19 Vaccine in Long-Term Care Facility Residents and Healthcare Workers – a Danish Cohort Study," medRxiv preprint, March 9, 2021, https://www.medrxiv.org/content/10.1101/2021.03.08.21252200v1

145   Scientific Advisory Group for Emergencies, "Eighty-Third SAGE Meeting on COVID-19," March 11, 2021, https://assets.publishing.service.gov.uk/government/uploads/system/uploads/attachment_data/file/975918/S1141_SAGE_83_minutes.pdf

146   Ibid., 41.

147   Day, "Warnings."

148   Isabel Kershner, "Israel's Push to Vaccinate Raises Host of Legal, Moral and Ethical Questions," *New York Times*, February 19, 2021, A6.

149   Azmi Haroun and Hilary Bruek, "CDC Director Says Data 'Suggests That Vaccinated People Do Not Carry the Virus,'" *Business Insider*, March 30, 2021, https://www.businessinsider.com/cdc-director-data-vaccinated-people-do-not-carry-covid-19-2021-3

150   Pfizer, "Pfizer and BioNTech Confirm High Efficacy and No Serious Safety Concerns through up to Six Months following Second Dose

in Updated Topline Analysis of Landmark COVID-19 Vaccine Study," April 1, 2021, https://investors.pfizer.com/Investors/News/news-details/2021/Pfizer-and-BioNTech-Confirm-High-Efficacy-and-No-Serious-Safety-Concerns-Through-Up-to-Six-Months-Following-Second-Dose-in-Updated-Topline-Analysis-of-Landmark-COVID-19-Vaccine-Study-04-01-2021/default.aspx

151   Stephen J. Thomas et al., "Six Month Safety and Efficacy of the BNT162b2 mRNA COVID-19 Vaccine," medRxiv preprint, July 28, 2021, https://www.medrxiv.org/content/10.1101/2021.07.28.21261159v1

152   Patricia Kime, "Pentagon Tracking 14 Cases of Heart Inflammation in Troops after COVID-19 Shots," military.com, April 26, 2021, https://www.military.com/daily-news/2021/04/26/pentagon-tracking-14-cases-of-heart-inflammation-troops-after-covid-19-shots.html

153   Derek Lowe, "Spike Protein Behavior," *Science Blogs*, May 4, 2021, https://www.science.org/content/blog-post/spike-protein-behavior

154   Ibid.

155   CDC, "Meeting of the Advisory Committee on Immunization Practices (ACIP)," May 12, 2021.

156   Berkley Lovelace, Jr., "CDC OKs Pfizer's Covid Vaccine for Use in Adolescents, Clearing the Way for Shots to Begin Thursday," CNBC, May 12, 2021, https://www.cnbc.com/2021/05/12/pfizer-covid-vaccine-cdc-panel-endorses-for-use-in-kids-12-to-15.html

157   Jennie S. Lavine, Ottar Bjornstadt, and Rustom Antia, "Vaccinating Children against SARS-CoV-2," *BMJ* 202;373n117

158   CDC, "COVID-19 VaSt Work Group Report," May 17, 2021, https://www.cdc.gov/vaccines/acip/work-groups-vast/report-2021-05-17.html?CDC_AA_refVal=https%3A%2F%2Fwww.cdc.gov%2Fvaccines%2Facip%2Fwork-groups-vast%2Ftechnical-report-2021-05-17.html

159   Cincinnati Children's, "Myocarditis in Children," updated April 2019, https://www.cincinnatichildrens.org/health/m/myocarditis

160   MSNBC, "Transcript: All in One with Chris Hayes, 5/17/21," May 17, 2021, https://www.msnbc.com/transcripts/transcript-all-chris-hayes-5-17-21-n1267740

161   Roxana Bruno et al., "SARS-CoV-2 Mass Vaccination: Urgent Questions on Vaccine Safety That Demand Answers from International Health Agencies, Regulatory Authorities, Governments, and Vaccine Developers," May 18, 2021.

162   Hanna Ziady, "Covid Vaccine Profits Mint 9 New Pharma Billionaires," Reuters, May 21, 2021, https://www.cnn.com/2021/05/21/business/covid-vaccine-billionaires/index.html

163   Internet Archive Wayback Machine, "Vaccine," November 5, 2020, https://web.archive.org/web/20201105154809/https://www.merriam-webster.com/dictionary/vaccine

164   Merriam-Webster, "Vaccine," accessed May 17, 2022, https://www.merriam-webster.com/dictionary/vaccine

165   Sudiksha Kochi, "Fact Check: Missing Context in Claim That Merriam-Webster Changed 'Vaccine' Definition," *USA Today*, November 30, 2021, https://www.usatoday.com/story/news/factcheck/2021/11/30/fact-check-merriam-webster-changed-vaccine-definition-accuracy/6354415001/

166   Linda Wastila et al., "Citizen Petition," June 1, 2021, https://www.regulations.gov/docket/FDA-2021-P-0521/document

167   Shari Roan, "Swine Flu 'Debacle' of 1976 Is Recalled," *Los Angeles Times*, April 27, 2009, https://www.latimes.com/archives/la-xpm-2009-apr-27-sci-swine-history27-story.html

168   Linda Wastila et al., "Why We Petitioned the FDA to Refrain from Fully Approving Any Covid-19 Vaccine This Year," *BMJ Blogs*, June 8, 2021, https://blogs.bmj.com/bmj/2021/06/08/why-we-petitioned-the-fda-to-refrain-from-fully-approving-any-covid-19-vaccine-this-year/

169   Peter Doshi, "Covid-19 Vaccines in Children: Be Careful," UMB Digital Archives, June 10, 2021, https://archive.hshsl.umaryland.edu/handle/10713/16065

170   Tom Shimabukuro, "COVID-19 Vaccine Safety Updates," June 10, 2021, https://cdc.gov/coronavirus

171   Kyle LaHucik, "He Authorized Moderna's Vaccine 6 Months Ago. Now Ex-FDA Chief Hahn Joins Biotech's Backer," *Fierce Biotech*, July 14, 2021, https://www.fiercebiotech.com/biotech/six-months-after-granting-moderna-covid-19-eua-ex-fda-commish-joins-biotech-s-founding

172   Pfizer, "US FDA Grants Priority Review for the Biologics License Application for Pfizer-BioNTech COVID-19 Vaccine," July 16, 2021, https://cdn.pfizer.com

173   White House, "Press Briefing by Press Secretary Jen Psaki," July 16, 2021, https://www.whitehouse.gov/briefing-room/press-briefings/2021/07/16/press-briefing-by-press-secretary-jen-psaki-july-16-2021/

174   Zolan Kanno-Youngs and Cecilia Kang, "'They're Killing People': Biden Denounces Social Media for Virus Disinformation," *New York Times*, July 16, 2021.

175   White House, "Remarks by President Biden in a CNN Town Hall with Don Lemon," July 22, 2021, https://www.whitehouse.gov/briefing-room/speeches-remarks/2021/07/22/remarks-by-president-biden-in-a-cnn-town-hall-with-don-lemon/

176   i24NEWS, "Vaccine 39% Effective at Halting Virus Transmission, 91% against Serious Illness, Israel's Health Ministry Says," July 22, 2021, https://www.i24news.tv/en/news/coronavirus/1626980447-vaccine-39-effective-at-halting-virus-transmission-91-against-serious-illness-israel-s-health-ministry-says

177   Yair Goldberg, et al., "Waning Immunity after the BNT162b Vaccine in Israel," *New England Journal of Medicine* 385, no. 4 (December 9, 2021), https:doi.org/10.1056/NEJMoa2114228

178   i24NEWS, "This is Not the Time to Debate Vaccines but to Get Them, Israel's Bennett Tells Refusniks," July 22, 2021, https://www.i24news.tv/en/news/israel/1626976195-this-is-not-the-time-to-debate-vaccines-but-to-get-them-israel-s-bennett-tells-refuseniks

179   Catherine M. Brown, et al., "Outbreak of SARS-CoV-2 Infections, Including COVID-19 Vaccine Breakthrough Infections, Associated with

Large Public Gatherings – Barnstable County, Massachusetts, July 2021," *Morbidity and Mortality Weekly Report* 70, (July 30, 2021), https://www. cdc.gov/mmwr/volumes/70/wr/mm7031e2.htm

180   Mark Joyella, "CNN's Don Lemon on the Unvaccinated: 'Their Behavior Is Idiotic and Nonsensical,'" *Forbes*, July 24, 2021, https://www.forbes. com/sites/markjoyella/2021/07/24/cnns-don-lemon-on-the-unvaccinat-ed-their-behavior-is-idiotic-and-nonsensical/?sh=752cd52f4b76

181   David Olive, "Vaccine Resisters Are Lazy and Irresponsible – We Need Vaccine Passports Now to Protect the Rest of Us," *Toronto Star*, July 30, 2021, https://www.thestar.com/business/opinion/2021/07/30/ we-need-a-national-vaccination-passport-recognized-through-out-the-world.html

182   Jessica Valenti, "Unvaxxed, Unmasked, and Putting Our Kids at Risk," *New York Times*, August 1, 2021.

183   Chris Hauser, "Get a COVID-19 Vaccine or Face Prison, Judge Order in Probation Cases," *New York Times,* August 9, 2021.

184   Mark Segraves, "DC Offers Free Beer at Kennedy Center for Getting Vaccine," NBC News Washington, May 4, 2021, https://www.nbcwash-ington.com/news/coronavirus/dc-offers-free-beer-at-kennedy-center-for-getting-vaccine/2661082/; CBS News, "New York City Mayor Bill DeBlasio Promotes a New Incentive to Get Vaccinated: Shake Shack," May 13, 2021, https://www.cbsnews.com/video/new-york-city-mayor-bill-de-blasio-covid-19-vaccine-free-shake-shack/#x; Jessica Dickler, "Krispy Kreme Doubles Its Free Donut Incentive for Vaccinations," CNBC, August 30, 2021, https://www.cnbc.com/2021/08/30/krispy-kreme-doubles-its-free-doughnut-incentive-for-vaccinations.html; Jesus Jiménez, "Washington State Allows for Free Marijuana with COVID-19 Vaccine," *New York Times,* June 7, 2021.

185   Ethan Alter, "Arnold Schwarzenegger's 'Screw Your Freedom' Remark Leads to a Sponsorship Loss," Yahoo Entertainment, August 24, 2021, https://www.yahoo.com/entertainment/arnold-schwarzenegger-sponsor-ship-loss-184606881.html

186   FDA, "What Is Gene Therapy?" page last updated July 25, 2018, accessed May 16, 2022, https://www.fda.gov/vaccines-blood-biologics/cellular-gene-therapy-products/what-gene-therapy

187   Pfizer, "Board Member: James C. Smith," 2022, https://www.pfizer.com/people/leadership/board_of_directors/james_smith

188   Pfizer, "Pfizer and BioNTech Announce Submission of Initial Data to US FDA to Support Booster Dose of COVID-19 Vaccine," August 16, 2021, https://www.pfizer.com/news/press-release/press-release-detail/pfizer-and-biontech-announce-submission-initial-data-us-fda

189   Pfizer, "Pfizer-BioNTech COVID-19 Vaccine Comirnaty™ Receives Full US FDA Approval for Individuals 16 Years and Older," August 23, 2021, https://www.pfizer.com/news/press-release/press-release-detail/pfizer-biontech-covid-19-vaccine-comirnatyr-receives-full

190   FDA, "FDA Approves First Covid-19 Vaccine," August 23, 2021, https://www.fda.gov/news-events/press-announcements/fda-approves-first-covid-19-vaccine

191   Gareth Iacobucci, "Covid-19: FDA Set to Grant Full Approval to Pfizer Vaccine without Public Discussion of Data," *BMJ* 2021;374n2086

192   Peter Doshi, "Does the FDA Think These Data Justify the First Full Approval of a COVID-19 Vaccine?" *BMJ Blogs*, August 23, 2021, https://blogs.bmj.com/bmj/2021/08/23/does-the-fda-think-these-data-justify-the-first-full-approval-of-a-covid-19-vaccine/

193   Thomas et al., "Safety and Efficacy."

194   Kasen K. Riemersma et al., "Shedding of Infectious SARS-CoV-2 Despite Vaccination," medRxiv preprint, August 24, 2021, https://www.medrxiv.org/content/10.1101/2021.07.31.21261387v4

195   *Toronto Star*, "Simmering Divide over Who Isn't Vaccinated," August 26, 2021.

196   Sophia Tulp, "Experts Say Changes to CDC's Vaccination Definition Are Normal," Associated Press, February 9, 2022, https://apnews.com/article/fact-checking-976069264061

197 Dominick Reuter, "Fauci Says US Is 'Perilously Close' to Doctors Having to Prioritize People for ICU Beds," *Business Insider*, September 6, 2021, https://www.businessinsider.com/fauci-says-us-doctors-may-have-to-prioritize-icu-beds-2021-9

198 Timothy Bella, "Jimmy Kimmel Suggests Hospitals Shouldn't Treat Unvaccinated People," *Washington Post*, September 8, 2021.

199 Daniel Krepps, "Howard Stern to 'Imbecile' Anti-Vaxxers: 'Go F—k Yourself,'" *Rolling Stone*, September 9, 2021, https://www.rollingstone.com/culture/culture-news/howard-stern-anti-vaxxers-go-fuck-yourself-1222672/

200 Robby Soave, "CNN's Leana Wen: The Unvaccinated Should Not Be Allowed to Leave Their Homes," *Reason*, September 10, 2021, https://reason.com/2021/09/10/cnn-leana-wen-unvaccinated-travel-outdoor-ban/

201 Lindsay Kornick, "Liberals Cheer on Biden's Anger toward the Unvaccinated During COVID Address," Fox News, September 9, 2021, https://www.foxnews.com/media/intense-mixed-reactions-biden-anger-at-the-unvaccinated

202 Darragh Roche, "Members of Congress and Their Staff Are Exempt from Biden's Vaccine Mandate," *Newsweek*, September 10, 2021, https://www.newsweek.com/members-congress-staff-exempt-biden-covid-vaccine-mandate-1627859

203 Asher Notheis, "Don Lemon Says Unvaccinated Should be 'Shunned' or 'Left Behind,'" Yahoo News, September 16, 2021, https://www.yahoo.com/video/don-lemon-says-unvaccinated-people-175300636.html

204 Bill and Melinda Gates Foundation, "Committed Grants: CNN.com," September 2020, https://www.gatesfoundation.org/about/committed-grants/2020/09/inv004478

205 Keith Speights, "Stocks the Bill & Melinda Gates Foundation Is Betting on," September 24, 2020, https://www.fool.com/investing/2020/09/24/4-coronavirus-vaccine-stocks-the-bill-melinda-gate/

206 Tom Rosenstiel et al., "Charting New Ground: The Ethical Terrain of Nonprofit Journalism," American Press Institute, April 20, 2016, https://www.americanpressinstitute.org/publications/reports/nonprofit-news/

207 FDA, "FDA Authorizes Booster Dose of Pfizer-BioNTech COVID-19 Vaccine for Certain Populations," September 22, 2022, https://www.fda.gov/news-events/press-announcements/fda-authorizes-booster-dose-pfizer-biontech-covid-19-vaccine-certain-populations

208 S.V. Subramanian and Akhil Kumar, "Increases in COVID-19 are Unrelated to Levels of Vaccination Across 68 Counties and 2947 Counties in the United States," *European Journal of Epidemiology* 36, (2021): 1237-1240, https://doi.org/10.1007/s10654-021-00808-7

209 Peter Roger Breggin and Ginger Ross Breggin, *COVID-19 and the Global Predators: We Are the Prey* (Ithaca: Lake Edge Press, September 30, 2021).

210 FDA, "Coronavirus (COVID-19) Update: FDA Takes Additional Actions on the Use of a Booster Dose for COVID-19 Vaccine," October 20, 2021, https://www.fda.gov/news-events/press-announcements/coronavirus-covid-19-update-fda-takes-additional-actions-use-booster-dose-covid-19-vaccines

211 FDA, "Vaccines and Related Biological Products Advisory Committee Meeting," October 26, 2021.

212 FDA, "Vaccines and Related Biological Products Advisory Committee – 10/26/2021," YouTube, October 26, 2021, https://www.youtube.com/watch?v=laaL0_xKmmA&t=24733s

213 New York City, "Mayor de Blasio Announces Vaccine Mandate for New York City Workers," October 20, 2021, https://www.nyc.gov/office-of-the-mayor/news/698-21/mayor-de-blasio-vaccine-mandate-new-york-city-workforce

214 FDA, "FDA Authorizes Pfizer-BioNTech COVID-19 Vaccine for Emergency Use in Children 5 Through 11 Years of Age," October 29, 2021, https://www.fda.gov/news-events/press-announcements/fda-authorizes-pfizer-biontech-covid-19-vaccine-emergency-use-children-5-through-11-years-age

215   Paul D. Thacker, "Revelations of Poor Practices at a Contract Research Company Helping to Carry out Pfizer's Pivotal Covid-19 Vaccine Trial Raise Questions about Data Integrity and Regulatory Oversight," *BMJ* 2021;375:n2635

216   Dean Miller, "Fact Check: The BMJ Did NOT Reveal Disqualifying and Ignored Reports of Flaws in Pfizer COVID-19 Vaccine Trials," Lead Stories, November 10, 2021, https://leadstories.com/hoax-alert/2021/11/fact-check-british-medical-journal-did-not-reveal-disqualifying-and-ignored-reports-of-flaws-in-pfizer-vaccine-trial.html

217   Jenna Greene, "Wait What? FDA Wants 55 Years to Process FOIA Request Over Vaccine Data," Reuters, November 18, 2021, https://www.reuters.com/legal/government/wait-what-fda-wants-55-years-process-foia-request-over-vaccine-data-2021-11-18/

218   Jenna Greene, "We'll All Be Dead before FDA Releases Full COVID Vaccine Records, Plaintiffs Say," Reuters, December 14, 2021, https://www.reuters.com/legal/government/well-all-be-dead-before-fda-releases-full-covid-vaccine-record-plaintiffs-say-2021-12-13/

219   United States Department of Health and Human Services, "Secretarial Directive on Availability of Booster Doses of COVID-19 Vaccines," November 21, 2021, https://www.hhs.gov/sites/default/files/secretarial-directive-availability-booster-doses-covid-19-vaccines.pdf

220   Philip R. Krause and Luciana Borio, "The Biden Administration Has Been Sidelining Vaccine Experts," *Washington Post*, December 19, 2021, B2.

221   World Health Organization, "Classification of Omicron (B.1.1.529): SARS-Cov-2 Variant of Concern," November 26, 2021, https://www.who.int/news/item/26-11-2021-classification-of-omicron-(b.1.1.529)-sars-cov-2-variant-of-concern

222   CDC, "SARS-CoV-2 B.1.1.529 (Omicron) Variant – United States, December 1-8, 2021," *Morbidity and Mortality Weekly Report* 70, no. 50 (December 17, 2021): 1731-1734, December 17, 2021, https://www.cdc.gov/mmwr/volumes/70/wr/mm7050e1.htm

223 United States Department of Health and Human Services, "Secretarial Directive on Availability of Booster Doses of COVID-19 Vaccines," December 10, 2021, https://www.hhs.gov/sites/default/files/secretarial-directive availability-booster-doses-covid-19-vaccines-december-2021.pdf

224 Krause and Borio, "Experts," B2.

225 Allie Malloy and Maegan Vazquez, "Biden Warns of Winter of 'Severe Illness and Death' for Unvaccinated Due to Omicron," CNN, December 16, 2021, https://www.cnn.com/2021/12/16/politics/joe-biden-warning-winter/index.html

226 Fiona Goodlee and Kamran Abbasi, "Open Letter to Mark Zuckerberg," *BMJ*, December 17, 2021, https://www.bmj.com/content/375/bmj.n2635/rr-80

227 Dean Miller, "Lead Stories Response to BMJ Open Letter Objecting to a Lead Stories Fact Check," Lead Stories, December 18, 2021, https://leadstories.com/analysis/2021/12/lead-stories-response-to-a-bmjcom-open-letter-objecting-to-a-lead-stories-fact-check.html

228 Sherry Gay Stolberg and Rebecca Robbins, "Moderna Moves for Total Credit in Vaccine Patent," *New York Times*, November 10, 2021.

229 *Nature*, "What the Moderna-NIH COVID Vaccine Patent Fight Means for Research," November 30, 2021, https://doi.org/10.1038/d41586-021-03535-x

230 New York City, "Mayor de Blasio Announces Vaccine Mandate for Private Sector Workers, and Major Expansions to Nation-Leading 'Key to NYC Program,'" December 6, 2021, https://www.nyc.gov/office-of-the-mayor/news/807-21/mayor-de-blasio-vaccine-mandate-private-sector-workers-major-expansions-to

231 Charles M. Blow, "I'm Furious at the Unvaccinated," *New York Times*, December 8, 2021.

232 Andrew Neil, "It's Time to Punish Britain's Five Million Vaccine Refuseniks," *Daily Mail*, December 9, 2021, https://www.dailymail.co.uk/debate/article-10294225/Its-time-punish-Britains-five-million-vaccine-refuseniks-says-ANDREW-NEIL.html

233 Anne McElvoy, "The Unvaccinated Have Become a Lethal Liability We Can Ill-Afford," *Evening Standard*, December 14, 2021, https://www.standard.co.uk/comment/covid-unvaccinated-omicron-vaccine-passports-b971877.html

234 Anonymous, "I Am Struggling to Understand Why Patients Decide Not to Get the Covid Vaccine," *BMJ* 2021;375:n3152

235 David Healy, "A Reason for Hesitancy," *BMJ*, December 27, 2021, https://www.bmj.com/content/375/bmj.n3152/rr

236 Dave Naylor, "Trudeau Calls the Unvaccinated Racist and Misogynistic Extremists," *Western Standard News*, December 29, 2021, https://www.westernstandard.news/news/trudeau-calls-the-unvaccinated-racist-and-misogynistic-extremists/article_a3bacece-2e14-5b8c-bf37-eddd672205f3.html

237 Bernard La Scola et al., "Viral RNA Load as Determined by Cell Culture as a Management Tool for Discharge of SARS-CoV-2 Patients from Infectious Disease Wards," *European Journal of Clinical Microbiology and Infectious Diseases* 39, no. 6 (June 2020): 1059-1061, https://doi.org/10.1007/s10096-020-03913-9

238 Rita Jaafar et al., "Correlation between 3790 Quantitative Polymerase Chain Reaction-Positive Samples and Positive Cell Cultures, Including 1941 Severe Acute Respiratory Syndrome Coronavirus 2 Isolates," *Clinical Infectious Diseases* 72, no. 11 (June 1, 2021): e921, https://doi.org/10.1093/ciaa1491

239 Apoorva Mandavilli, "Your Coronavirus Test Is Positive. Maybe It Shouldn't Be," *New York Times*, August 29, 2020.

240 Accessed 4 May 2021, link broken as of 13 June 2022, https://wwwn.cdc.gov/nndss/conditions/coronavirus-disease-2019-covid-19/case-definition/2020/08/05/

241 CDC, "Weekly Updates by Select Demographic and Geographic Characteristics: Provisional Death Counts for Coronavirus Disease 2019 (COVID-19): Comorbidities and Other Conditions," June 2, 2022, https://www.cdc.gov/nchs/nvss/vsrr/covid_weekly/index.htm#Comorbidities

242   *Spectator*, "Hospitals Get Paid More to List Patients as COVID-19 and Three Times as Much if Patient Goes on Ventilator," April 9, 2020, https://thespectator.info/2020/04/09/hospitals-get-paid-more-to-list-patients-as-covid-19-and-three-times-as-much-if-the-patient-goes-on-ventilator-video/?utm_source=wnd&utm_medium=wnd&utm_campaign=syndicated

243   Federal Emergency Management Agency, "Funeral Assistance FAQ," July 20, 2021, https://www.fema.gov/disaster/coronavirus/economic/funeral-assistance/faq

244   *Spectator*, "Hospitals."

245   Schematic mechanism of PCR. Enzoklop, CC BY-SA 4.0 <https://creativecommons.org/licenses/by-sa/4.0>, via Wikimedia Commons

246   World Health Organization, "COVID-19 Vaccines Advice," updated April 13, 2022, https://www.who.int/emergencies/diseases/novel-coronavirus-2019/covid-19-vaccines/advice

247   CDC, "Frequently Asked Questions about COVID-19 Vaccination," updated July 11, 2022, https://www.cdc.gov/coronavirus/2019-ncov/vaccines/faq.html

248   Martin Kulldorff, Sunetra Gupta, and Jay Bhattacharya, "Great Barrington Declaration," October 4, 2020, https://gbdeclaration.org/

249   *Wall Street Journal*, "How Fauci and Collins Shut Down Covid Debate: They Worked with Media to Trash the Great Barrington Declaration," December 21, 2020.

250   David Gorski, "COVID-19 Deniers Follow the Path Laid Down by Creationists, HIV/AIDS Denialists, and Climate Science Deniers," Science-Based Medicine, October 12, 2020, https://sciencebasedmedicine.org/great-barrington-declaration/

251   Kristina Alexanderson et al., "John Snow Memorandum," October 14, 2020, https://www.johnsnowmemo.com/john-snow-memo.html

252   John Snow, "Cholera and the Water Supply in the South Districts of London in 1854," *Journal of Public Health and Sanitary Review* 2, no. 7 (October 1856): 239-257.

253　Noah Kojima and Jeffrey D. Klausner, "Protective Immunity after Recovery from SARS-CoV-2 Infection," *Lancet Infectious Diseases* 22, no. 1 (January 2022): 12-14, https://doi.org/10.1016/S1473-3099(21)00676-9

254　Block, "Natural Immunity," 3.

255　Ibid., 2.

256　"Sivan Gazit et al., "Comparing SARS-CoV-2 Natural Immunity to Vaccine-Induced Immunity: Reinfections versus Breakthrough Infections," medRxiv preprint, August 25, 2021, https://doi.org10.1101/2021.08.24.21262415

257　Alexander G. Mathioudakis et al., "Self-Reported Real-World Safety and Reactogenicity of COVID-19 Vaccines: A Vaccine Recipient Survey," *Life*, 11, no. 249 (2021): 1-13, https://doi.org/10.3390/life11030249

258　Yuanyuan Dong et al., "Epidemiology of COVID-19 among Children in China," *Pediatrics* 2020;145(6):e20200702

259　FAIR Health, "Risk Factors for COVID-19 Mortality among Privately Insured Patients," November 11, 2020, https://www.fairhealth.org/publications/whitepapers

260　Sunil S. Bhopal et al., "Children and Young People Remain at Low Risk of COVID-19 Mortality," *Lancet: Child and Adolescent Health* 5, March 10, 2021, https://doi.org/10.1016/S2352-4642(21)00066-3

261　Daniela Say et al. "Post-Acute COVID-19 Outcomes in Children with Mild and Asymptomatic Disease," *Lancet: Child and Adolescent Health* 5, (June 2021): 22-23, https://doi.org/10.1016/S2352-4642(21)00124-3

262　Claire Smith et al., "Deaths in Children and Young People in England Following SARS-CoV-2 During the First Pandemic Year: A National Study Using Linked Mandatory Child Death Reporting Data," medRxiv preprint, July 8, 2021, https://www.medrxiv.org/content/10.1101/2021.07.07.21259779v1

263　European Centre for Disease Prevention and Control, "COVID-19 in Children and the Role of School in Transmission – Second Update," July

8, 2021, https://www.ecdc.europa.eu/en/publications-data/children-and-school-settings-covid-19-transmission

264 Joe Hernandez, "Nearly 94,000 Kids Got COVID-19 Last Week. They Were 15% of All New Cases," National Public Radio, August 10, 2021, https://www.npr.org/sections/coronavirus-live-up-dates/2021/08/10/1026375608/nearly-94-000-kids-got-covid-19-last-week-they-were-15-of-all-new-infections

265 Kevin Ng et al., "Preexisting and de Novo Humoral Immunity to SARS-CoV-2 in Humans," *Science* 370, (December 11, 2020): 1339-1343, https://doi.org/10.101126/science.abe1107

266 Puneet Misra et al., "Serological Prevalence of SARS-CoV-2 Antibody among Children and Young Age (Between Age 2-17 Years) Group in India: An Interim Result from a Large Multicentric Population-Based Seroepidemiological Study," medRxiv preprint, June 16, 2021, https://www.medrxiv.org/content/10.1101/2021.06.15.21258880v1

267 Margaret Menge, "Indiana Life Insurance CEO Says Deaths Are up 40% among People Ages 18-64," Center Square, January 1, 2022, https://www.thecentersquare.com/indiana/indiana-life-insurance-ceo-says-deaths-are-up-40-among-people-ages-18-64/article_71473b12-6b1e-11ec-8641-5b2c06725e2c.html

268 Ali Swenson, "Vaccines Didn't Cause Increase in Deaths and Life Insurance Payouts," Associated Press, January 10, 2022, https://apnews.com/article/fact-checking-692312045885?utm_campaign=SocialFlow&utm_medium=APFactCheck&utm_source=Twitter

269 Madison Czopek, "No, COVID-19 Vaccines Aren't Responsible for an Increase in Deaths," PolitiFact, February 1, 2022, https://www.politifact.com/factchecks/2022/feb/11/blog-posting/no-covid-19-vaccines-arent-responsible-increase-de/

270 Angie Drobnic Holan, "Poynter Institute Announces Initiative to Fact-Check Claims about Global Health and Development," PolitiFact, January 25, 2016, https://www.politifact.com/article/2016/jan/25/poynter-institute-announces-initiative-fact-check-/

271 Olivier Beaumont, David Doukhan, Pauline Théveniaud, Henri Vernet, and Marcelo Wesfried, "Europe, Vaccination, Présidentielle … Emmanuel Macron Se Livre à nos Lecteurs," *Le Parisien*, January 4, 2022, https://www.leparisien.fr/politique/europe-vaccination-presidentielle-emmanu-el-macron-se-livre-a-nos-lecteurs-04-01-2022-2KVQ3ESNSREABMT-DWR25OMGWEA.php?ts=1641326582881

272 Michael Hiltzik, "Mocking Anti-Vaxxers' COVID Deaths Is Ghoulish, Yes – But May Be Necessary," *Los Angeles Times*, January 10, 2022.

273 James McAuley, "Macron is Right: It's Time to Make Life a Living Hell for Anti-Vaxxers," *Washington Post*, January 11, 2022.

274 Heather Mallick, "The Unvaccinated Cherish Their Freedom to Harm Others. How Can We Ever Forgive Them?" *Toronto Star*, January 15, 2022, https://www.thestar.com/politics/political-opinion/2022/01/15/the-unvaccinated-cherish-their-freedom-to-harm-others-how-can-we-ever-forgive-them.html

275 Evan Dyer, "Public Outrage over the Unvaccinated is Driving a Crisis in Bioethics," CBC News, January 22, 2022, https://www.cbc.ca/news/politics/pandemic-covid-vaccine-triage-omicron-1.6319844

276 Polly Hudson, "As Covid Restrictions Ease, It's Time to Get Tough on Anti-Vaxxers," *Mirror*, January 25, 2022, https://www.mirror.co.uk/news/uk-news/as-covid-restrictions-ease-its-26046616?fbclid=IwAR30KhFu-rOXa4sE0l79TBPPfL5IJLZ9JylvUShS5daW_wHciLkYqcIR14ak

277 Heba Altarawneh et al., "Protection by Prior Infection against SARS-CoV-2 Reinfection with the Omicron Variant," medRxiv preprint, January 6, 2022, https://www.medrxiv.org/content/10.1101/2022.01.05.22268782v1

278 Peter Doshi, Fiona Goodlee, and Kamran Abbasi, "Covid-19 Vaccines and Treatments: We Must Have Raw Data, Now," *BMJ* 2022;376:o102

279 David Healy, "The Evidence That Counts for the FDA," January 19, 2022, https://davidhealy.org/the-evidence-that-counts-for-fda/

280 David Healy, "The Evidence That Counts for Us," January 26, 2022, https://davidhealy.org/the-evidence-that-counts-for-us/

281   Ed Payne, "Fact Check: DOD Whistleblowers 'Mind Blowing COVID Vaccine Injury Numbers' Were Not Based on Accurate Data, Pentagon Says," Lead Stories, February 1, 2022, https://leadstories.com/hoax-alert/2022/02/fact-check-dod-whistleblowers-mind-blowing-covid-vaccine-injury-numbers-were-not-based-on-accurate-data.html?fbclid=IwAR05_--On8kEKHdfxSf130eN5J7sGY3AloIK3u3xCoVg0SZmWt6hz9Rwbcs

282   Pfizer, "Pfizer and BioNTech Initiate Rolling Submission for Emergency Use Authorization of Their COVID-19 Vaccine in Children 6 Months through 4 Years of Age Following Request from U.S. FDA," February 1, 2022, https://www.pfizer.com/news/press-release/press-release-detail/pfizer-and-biontech-initiate-rolling-submission-emergency

283   Ibid.

284   Ibid.

285   Sharon LaFraniere and Noah Weiland, "Pfizer Asks FDA to Clear 2 Vaccine Doses for Young Children as a Start," *New York Times*, February 1, 2022, A10.

286   Ibid.

287   Ibid.

288   Diego Montano, "Frequency and Associations of Adverse Reactions of COVID-19 Vaccines Reported to Pharmacovigilance Systems in the European Union and the United States," *Frontiers in Public Health* 9, Article 756633 (February 3, 2022): 1-16, https://doi.org/10.3389/fpubh.2021.756633

289   Apoorva Mandavilli, "CDC Data Suggests Boosters' Protection against Severe COVID-19 Plunges after 4 Months," *New York Times*, February 11, 2022.

290   Sharon LaFraniere and Noah Weiland, "FDA Delays Shots for Those under Age of 5," *New York Times*, February 12, 2022, A1.

291   Zachary Stieber, "Pfizer Trial Whistleblower Presses forward with Lawsuit without Government Help," *Epoch Times*, February 14, 2022, https://www.theepochtimes.com/mkt_app/exclusive-pfizer-tri-

al-whistleblower-presses-forward-with-lawsuit-without-us-govern-ments-help_4277153.html

292   Associated Press, "NYC Fires More Than 1,000 Workers over Vaccine Mandate," *New York Times*, February 14, 2022.

293   Emma G. Fitzsimmons, "Nearly 3,000 NYC Workers Have a Day to Get Vaccinated or Be Fired," *New York Times*, February 11, 2022.

294   David Healy, "The Crack through Which Science Gets in," February 15, 2022, https://davidhealy.org/the-crack-through-which-the-science-gets-in/

295   David Healy, "Injuries in Vaccine Trials," February 22, 2022, https://davidhealy.org/injuries-in-vaccine-trials/

296   John Paul Tasker, "Trudeau Accuses Conservative MP's of Standing with 'People Who Wave Swastikas,'" CBC News, February 17, 2022, https://www.cbc.ca/news/politics/trudeau-conservative-swastikas-1.6354970

297   Fox News, "Trudeau Has Lost Control of the Situation: Canadian Parliament Member," February 17, 2022, https://www.youtube.com/watch?v=ooi9rfFUcic

298   Mathew Crawford, "Defining Away Vaccine Safety Signals 7: Fact Checkers Miss the Point," Substack, April 3, 2022, https://roundingthee-arth.substack.com/p/defining-away-vaccine-safety-signals-a10

299   UK Health Security Agency, "COVID-19 Vaccine Surveillance Report: Week 3," January 20, 2022.

300   Christian Holm Hansen et al., "Vaccine Effectiveness against SARS-CoV-2 Infection with the Omicron or Delta Variants Following a Two-Dose or Booster BNT162b2 mRNA Vaccination Series: A Danish Cohort Study," medRxiv preprint, December 22, 2021, https://www.medrxiv.org/content/10.1101/2021.12.20.21267966v2

301   HART Group, "Where's the Evidence for Waning Vaccine Immunity?" February 17, 2022, https://www.hartgroup.org/wheres-the-evi-dence-for-waning-vaccine-immunity/

302   HART Group, "Only a Fraction of the Population Is Susceptible to Each Variant," December 9, 2021, https://www.hartgroup.org/only-a-fraction-of-the-population-are-susceptible-to-each-variant/

303   HART Group, "Evidence."

304   Apoorva Mandavilli, "CDC Isn't Publishing Large Portion of COVID-19 Data It Collects," *New York Times*, February 20, 2022.

305   David Muoio, "How Many Employees Have Hospitals Lost to Vaccine Mandates? Here Are the Numbers So Far," *Fierce Healthcare*, February 22, 2022, https://www.fiercehealthcare.com/hospitals/how-many-employees-have-hospitals-lost-to-vaccine-mandates-numbers-so-far

306   Reuters, "Fact Check – Pages of Suspected Side Effects Released About Pfizer's COVID-19 Vaccine 'May Not Have Any Causal Relationship' to the Jab, Company Says," March 17, 2022, https://www.reuters.com/article/factcheck-coronavirus-pfizer/fact-check-pages-of-suspected-side-effects-released-about-pfizers-covid-19-vaccine-may-not-have-any-causal-relationship-to-the-jab-company-says-idUSL2N2VK1G1

307   Ewan Palmer, "What 'Pfizer Documents' Release Reveals," *Newsweek*, May 22, 2022, https://www.newsweek.com/pfizer-documents-vaccine-deaths-1703869

308   Sudiksha Kochi, "Fact Check: Claim Misrepresents Data from a Pfizer 2021 Report," *USA Today*, May 30, 2022, https://www.usatoday.com/story/news/factcheck/2022/05/30/fact-check-claim-misinterprets-data-2021-pfizer-report/9898129002/

309   Albert Bourla, *Moonshot* (New York: Harper Collins, March 8, 2022).

310   Hannah Devlin and Richard Adams, "Covid Resurgent across UK with Infections in over-70s at All-Time High," *Guardian*, March 18, 2022.

311   BBC, "Covid Vaccine: How Many People are Vaccinated in the UK?" March 4, 2022, https://www.bbc.com/news/health-55274833

312   Mathew Crawford, "Defining Away Vaccine Safety Signals 5: The DMED Data 'Glitch' Revealed?" Substack, March 22, 2022, https://roundingtheearth.substack.com/p/defining-away-vaccine-safety-signals-82f

313   CBS New York, "Mayor Adams Says Professional Athletes, Performers Now Exempt from Vaccine Mandate," March 24, 2022. https://www.cbsnews.com/newyork/live-updates/eric-adams-vaccine-mandate-pro-athletes-performers-kyrie-irving/

314   Gili Regev-Yochay et al., "Efficacy of a Fourth Dose of Covid-19 mRNA Vaccine against Omicron," *New England Journal of Medicine* 385, no. 14 (April 7, 2022): 1377-1380, https://doi.org/10.1056/NEJMc2202542

315   Sonja Elijah, "Was Pfizer's 95% Vaccine Efficacy Fraudulent All Along?" Substack, April 3, 2022, https://soniaelijah.substack.com/p/was-pfizers-95-vaccine-efficacy-fraudulent?s=r

316   Hannah Smith, "Post Claiming the Pfizer Vaccine Has Only a 12% Efficacy Rate Is Inaccurate," May 17, 2022, FullFact, https://fullfact.org/health/pfizer-vaccine-efficacy/

317   David Gorski, "The '12% Efficacy' Myth from the 'Pfizer Data Dump': The Latest Slasher Stat about COVID-19 Vaccines," Science-Based Medicine, May 9, 2022, https://sciencebasedmedicine.org/the-12-gambit-the-latest-slasher-stat-about-covid-19-vaccines/

318   Jeffrey Morris, "Do the Recent 80k Pages of Pfizer Documents Released Really Show Vaccine Efficacy Was Only 12%?" Covid-19 Data Science, May 5, 2022, https://www.covid-datascience.com/post/do-the-recent-80k-pages-of-pfizer-documents-released-really-show-vaccine-efficacy-was-only-12

319   Gorski, "Myth."

320   Ibid.

321   United States Department of Health and Human Services, "Secretarial Directive on Pediatric and Second COVID-19 Vaccine Booster Doses," May 23, 2022, https://www.hhs.gov/sites/default/files/secretarial-directive-on-pediatric-and-second-booster-dose.pdf

322   Phil Harper, "A Public Verification of Jikkyleaks," Substack, June 8, 2022, https://philharper.substack.com/p/a-public-verification-of-jikkyleaks

323   Dean Follmann, et al., "Anti-Nucleocapsid Antibodies following SARS-CoV-2 Infection in the Blinded Phase of the mRNA-1273

Covid-19 Vaccine Efficacy Clinical Trial," medRxiv preprint, April 19, 2022, https://www.medrxiv.org/content/10.1101/2022.04.18.22271936v1

324   United States Department of Health and Human Services, "Secretarial Directive on Pediatric COVID-19 Vaccines for Children 6 Months through 4/5 Years of Age," June 18, 2022.

325   Apoorva Mandavilli, "As Vaccines Arrive for the Youngest, Parents are Put on the Spot," *New York Times*, June 19, 2022, A1.

326   Sharon LaFraniere, "FDA May Move toward Updating Vaccines," *New York Times*, June 27, 2022.

327   Noah Weiland, "FDA Wants Covid Boosters Updated to Target Subvariants," *New York Times*, July 1, 2022, A13.

328   Lauren Leatherby, "How the BA.5 Subvariant May Affect the US," *New York Times*, July 8, 2022, A11.

329   Zachary Stieber, "Fauci, Other US Officials Served in Lawsuit over Alleged Collusion to Suppress Free Speech," *Epoch Times*, July 21, 2022, https://www.theepochtimes.com/fauci-other-us-officials-served-in-lawsuit-over-alleged-collusion-to-suppress-free-speech_4612827.html

330   Julie Boucau et al., "Duration of Shedding of Culturable Virus in SARS-CoV-2 Omicron (BA.1) Infection," *New England Journal of Medicine* 387, no. 3 (July 21, 2022): 275-277, https://www.nejm.org/doi/full/10.1056/nejmc2202092

331   Jason Lemon, "Video of Biden Saying Vaccinations Prevent COVID Resurfaces after Infection," *Newsweek*, July 21, 2022, https://www.newsweek.com/joe-biden-2021-video-saying-vaccinations-prevent-covid-resurfaces-1726900

332   YouTube, July 22, 2022, https://www.youtube.com/shorts/x8Sl9DORB_A

333   Zachary Stieber, "EXCLUSIVE: CDC Says It Performed Vaccine Safety Data Mining after Saying It Didn't," *Epoch Times*, July 23, 2022, https://www.theepochtimes.com/mkt_morningbrief/exclusive-cdc-says-it-performed-vaccine-safety-data-mining-after-saying-it-didnt_4617563.html

334   Jan Hoffman, "Few Parents Say They Plan to Vaccinate Young Children against Covid," *New York Times*, July 27, 2022, A17.

335   Noah Weiland, "Biden Administration Plant to Offer New Booster Shots in September," *New York Times*, July 29, 2022, A17.

336   *New York Times*, "Pfizer Continues Spree with $5.4 Billion Buy," August 9, 2022, B2.

337   Greta M. Masseti et al., "Summary of Guidance for Minimizing the Impact of COVID-19 in Individual Persons, Communities, and Health Care Systems – United States, August 2022," *Morbidity and Mortality Weekly Report* 71, (August 11, 2022): 1-9, https://www.cdc.gov/mmwr/volumes/71/wr/mm7133e1.htm

338   CDC, "Rates of COVID-19 Cases or Deaths by Age Groups and Vaccination Status and Second Booster Dose," updated October 21, 2022, https://data.cdc.gov/Public-Health-Surveillance/Rates-of-COVID-19-Cases-or-Deaths-by-Age-Group-and/d6p8-wqjm

339   Pfizer, "Statement from Pfizer Chairman and CEO Albert Bourla on Testing Positive for COVID-19," August 15, 2022, https://www.pfizer.com/news/announcements/statement-pfizer-chairman-and-ceo-albert-bourla-testing-positive-covid-19

340   Cedars Sinai, "New Data Show COVID-19 Vaccine Does Not Raise Stroke Risk," August 24, 2022, https://www.cedars-sinai.org/newsroom/new-data-shows-covid-19-vaccine-does-not-raise-stroke-risk/

341   Rebecca Robbins and Jenny Gross, "Moderna Sues Pfizer and BioNTech over Coronavirus Vaccine," *New York Times*, August 27, 2022, B1.

342   FDA, "Coronavirus (COVID-19) Update: FDA Authorizes Moderna, Pfizer-BioNTech COVID-19 Vaccines for Use as a Booster Dose," August 31, 2022.

343   Gretchen Vogel, "Omicron Booster Shots Are Coming – with Lots of Questions," *Science*, August 30, 2022, https://www.science.org/content/article/omicron-booster-shots-are-coming-lots-questions

344   FDA, "Booster."

345   Ibid.

346   Ibid.

347   Joseph Fraiman et al., "Serious Adverse Events of Special Interest following mRNA COVID-19 Vaccination in Randomized Trials in Adults," *Vaccine* 40, no. 40 (September 22, 2022): 5798-5805, https://doi.org/10.1016/j.vaccine.2022.08.036

348   United States Department of Health and Human Services, "Vaccine Side Effects," page last updated May 6, 2022, https://www.hhs.gov/immunization/basics/safety/side-effects/index.html

349   Rong-Gong Lin II, "Fears of More Long Covid, a 'Mass Disabling Event' as Variants Rip Through California," *Los Angeles Times*, July 26, 2022, https://www.latimes.com/california/story/2022-07-26/covid-19-reinfection-worsens-long-term-risk-for-death-fatigue-heart-disorders

350   Sumathi Reddy, "Over Two Million Americans Aren't Working Due to Long Covid; Brookings Institution Report Says the Loss of Work Translates into Roughly $170 Billion a Year in Lost Wages," *Wall Street Journal*, August 25, 2022, https://www.wsj.com/articles/over-2-million-americans-arent-working-due-to-long-covid-says-brookings-11661364528

351   Paul Garner, "For 7 Weeks I Have Been through a Roller Coaster of Ill Health, Extreme Emotions, and Utter Exhaustion," *BMJ Blogs*, May 5, 2020, https://blogs.bmj.com/bmj/2020/05/05/paul-garner-people-who-have-a-more-protracted-illness-need-help-to-understand-and-cope-with-the-constantly-shifting-bizarre-symptoms/

352   Ibid.

353   Felicity Callard and Elise Perego, "How and Why Patients Made Long Covid," *Social Science and Medicine* 268, (January 2021), https://doi.org/10.1016/j.socscimed2020.113426

354   Lara Keay, "Long-Term COVID Warning: ICU Doctor Reports Having Coronavirus Symptoms for Three Months," Sky News, June 25, 2020, https://news.sky.com/story/long-term-covid-warning-icu-doctor-reports-having-coronavirus-symptoms-for-three-months-12014361

355   Elizabeth Mahase, "Covid-19: What Do We Know About 'Long Covid?'" *BMJ* 2020;370:m2815

356   World Health Organization, "A Clinical Case Definition of Post COVID-19 Condition by a Delphi Consensus," October 6, 2021.

357   Hannah E. Davis et al., "Characterizing Long COVID in an International Cohort: 7 Months of Symptoms and Their Impact," *EClinical Medicine* 38, (2021), https://doi.org/10.1016/eclinm.2021.101019

358   Liane S. Canas et al., "Profiling Post-COVID Syndrome across Different Variants of SARS-CoV-2," medRxiv preprint, July 31, 2022, https://www.medrxiv.org/content/10.1101/2022.07.28.22278159v1

359   Anuradhaa Subramanian et al., "Symptoms and Risk Factors for Long COVID in Non-Hospitalized Adults," *Nature Medicine* 28, (2022): 1706-1714, https://www.nature.com/articles/s41591-022-01909-wdhaa

360   CDC, "Long COVID or Post-COVID Conditions," updated September 1, 2022, https://www.cdc.gov/coronavirus/2019-ncov/long-term-effects/index.html

361   Priya Venkatesan, "Do Vaccines Prevent Long COVID?" *Lancet Respiratory Medicine* 10, (January 22, 2022): e30, https://doi.org/10.1016/S2213-2600(22)00020-0

362   CDC, "Long COVID."

363   Will Stone, "Evidence Grows That Vaccines Lower the Risk of Getting Long COVID," National Public Radio, March 24, 2022, https://www.npr.org/sections/health-shots/2022/03/24/1088270403/long-covid-vaccines

364   Rong-Gong Lin II, "Fears."

365   Zeynep Tufeki, "There's Terrific News about the New Covid Boosters," *New York Times*, September 16, 2022, A22.

366   Ziyad Al-Aly, Benjamin Bowe, and Yan Xie, "Long COVID after Breakthrough SARS-CoV-2 Infection," *Nature Medicine* 28, no. 7 (July 2022): 1461-1467, https://doi.org/10.1038/s41591-022-01840-0

367   Aaron Kheriaty, "Our Lawsuit Uncovers Army of Federal Bureaucrats Coercing Social-Media Companies to Censor Speech," Substack, September 1, 2022, https://aaronkheriaty.substack.com/p/our-lawsuit-uncovers-army-of-federal

368   Suzanne Burdick, "'God Gave Us Two Arms – One for the Flu Shot, One for the COVID Shot,'" *Defender*, September 7, 2022, https://children-

shealthdefense.org/defender/ashish-jha-flu-shot-covid-shot-white-house-covid-response/

369   Kevin Bardosh et al., "Covid-19 Vaccine Boosters for Young Adults: A Risk-Benefit Assessment and Five Ethical Arguments against Vaccine Mandates at Universities," SSRN, September 12, 2022, https://papers.ssrn.com/sol3/papers.cfm?abstract_id=4206070

370   Jenin Younes, "The U.S. Government's Vast New Privatized Censorship Regime," *Tablet*, September 21, 2022, https://www.tabletmag.com/sections/arts-letters/articles/government-privatized-censorship-regime

371   Stephen Sorace, "Pfizer CEO Albert Bourla Tests Positive for COVID-19 for the Second Time in Less Than Two Months," Fox Business, September 25, 2022, https://www.foxbusiness.com/business-leaders/pfizer-ceo-albert-bourla-tests-positive-covid-19-second-time-less-than-2-months

372   Alison Edelman et al., "Association between Menstrual Cycle Length and Covid-19 Vaccination: Global, Retrospective Cohort Study of Prospectively Collected Data," *BMJMED* 2022;1:e000297

373   National Institutes of Health, "Study Confirms Link Between COVID-19 Vaccination and Temporary Increase in Menstrual Cycle Length," September 27, 2022, https://www.nih.gov/news-events/news-releases/study-confirms-link-between-covid-19-vaccination-temporary-increase-menstrual-cycle-length

374   Katherine M.N. Lee et al., "Characterizing Menstrual Bleeding Changes Occurring after SARS-CoV-2 Vaccination," medRxiv preprint, October 12, 2021, https://www.medrxiv.org/content/10.1101/2021.10.11.21 264863v1; Alexandra Alvergne et al., "COVID-19 Vaccination and Menstrual Cycle Changes: A United Kingdom (UK) Retrospective Case-Control Study," medRxiv preprint, December 6, 2021, https://www.medrxiv.org/content/10.1101/2021.11.23.21266709v3; Lill Trogstad et al., "Increased Occurrence of Menstrual Disturbances in 18- to 30-Year-Old Women after COVID-19 Vaccination," SSRN, January 14, 2022, https://papers.ssrn.com/sol3/papers.cfm?abstract_id=3998180

375   Lee et al., "Bleeding."

376   Naomi Wolf, *The Bodies of Others: Covid-19 and the War against the Human* (Fort Lauderdale: All Seasons Press, May 31, 2022).

377   Hung Fu Tseng, et al., "Effectiveness of mRNA-1273 against Infection and COVID-19 Hospitalization with SARS-CoC-2 Omicron Subvariants: BA.1, BA.2, BA.2.12.1, BA.4, and BA.5," medRxiv preprint, October 1, 2022, https://www.medrxiv.org/content/10.1101/2022.09.30.2 2280573v1.full.pdf

378   Florida Health, "Guidance for mRNA COVID-19 Vaccines," October 7, 2022. https://www.medrxiv.org/content/10.1101/2022.09.30.22280 573v1.full.pdf

379   David Gorski, "The State of Florida Spreads Antivaccine Disinformation Disguised as an Epidemiological Study," Science-Based Medicine, October 10, 2022, https://sciencebasedmedicine.org/the-state-of-florida-spreads-antivaccine-disinformation-disguised-as-an-epidemiological-study/

380   Frank Chung, "Pfizer Did Not Know Whether Covid Vaccine Stopped Transmission before Rollout, Executive Admits," news.com, October 13, 2022, https://www.news.com.au/technology/science/human-body/pfizer-did-not-know-whether-covid-vaccine-stopped-transmission-before-rollout-executive-admits/news-story/f307f28f794e173ac017a62784fec414

381   Ellen McCutchan, "Viral Pfizer 'Admission' Not What It Seems," RMIT FactLab, November 3, 2022, https://www.rmit.edu.au/news/factlab-meta/viral-pfizer--admission--not-what-it-seems?fbclid=IwAR2Xjry-TOddm9-ihUlyR17Suw8zbKCJ0qWA-9Zn0J3M7i7ssiLUOqYzVau0

382   Caitlin Tilley, "Moderna's CEO Admits Only the Vulnerable Need a COVID Booster and Likens the Virus to the Flu," *Daily Mail*, October 18, 2022, https://www.dailymail.co.uk/health/article-11327615/Modernas-CEO-admits-vulnerable-need-Covid-booster-shot.html

383   Reuters, "US CDC Advisers Approve Adding COVID Shots to Vaccine Schedule," October 20, 2022, https://www.reuters.com/world/us/us-cdc-advisers-approve-adding-covid-shots-vaccine-schedules-2022-10-20/

384   Julia Musto, "CDC Director Rochelle Walensky Tests Positive for COVID-19 Month after Getting Updated Booster Shot," Fox News,

October 22, 2022, https://www.foxnews.com/health/cdc-director-ro-chelle-walensky-tests-positive-covid-19-month-getting-updated-boost-er-shot

385 Katherine J. Wu, "The Worst Pediatric-Care Crisis in Decades," *Atlantic*, October 31, 2022.

386 Emily Oster, "Let's Declare a Pandemic Amnesty," *Atlantic*, October 31, 2022.

387 Katie Grimes, "California Doctors Sue Gov. Newsom and Medical Board over New Law Censoring Medical Advice," *California Globe*, November 2, 2022, https://californiaglobe.com/articles/california-doctors-sue-gov-newsom-and-medical-board-over-new-law-censoring-medical-advice/

388 Melissa Healy, "Are the Unvaccinated Still a Danger to the Rest of Us?" *Los Angeles Times*, November 3, 2022.

389 Mansur Shaheen, "Pfizer and Moderna Launch Trials to Track Whether Health Issues Arise YEARS after Getting Their Covid Vaccines," *Daily Mail*, November 14, 2022, https://www.dailymail.co.uk/health/article-11426007/Pfizer-Moderna-launch-trials-track-issues-arise-YEARS-get-ting-vaccines.html

390 Apoorva Mandavilli, "Will Covid Boosters Prevent Another Wave? Scientists Aren't So Sure," *New York Times*, November 19, 2022.

391 Yuxi Wang et al., "Understanding and Neutralising Covid-19 Misinfor-mation and Disinformation," *BMJ* 2022;379e070331

392 J.T. Stepleton, "Where There's Smoke, There's Big Tobacco... and Pharma and Telecom," followthemoney.org, September 9, 2017, https://www.followthemoney.org/research/blog/where-theres-smoke-theres-big-tobac-co-and-pharma-and-telecom

393 White House, "Press Briefing by Press Secretary Karine Jean-Pierre, COVID-19 Response Coordinator Dr. Ashish Jha, and Chief Medical Advisor Dr. Anthony Fauci," November 22, 2022, https://www.white-house.gov/briefing-room/press-briefings/2022/11/22/press-briefing-by-press-secretary-karine-jean-pierre-covid-19-response-coordinator-dr-ashish-jha-and-chief-medial-advisor-dr-anthony-fauci/

394   Lori Rozsa, "DeSantis Forms Panel to Counter CDC, a Move Decried by Health Professionals," *Washington Post*, December 13, 2022.

395   Philip Bump, "DeSantis Again Threatens Legal Action with an Eye on 2024," *Washington Post*, December 13, 2022.

396   Neil Jay Sehgal, et al., "The Association between COVID-19 Mortality and the County-Level Partisan Divide in the United States," *Health Affairs* 41, no 6 (June 2022), https://doi.org/10.1377/hlthaff.2022.00085

397   Isaac Arnsdorf, "DeSantis Reverses Himself on Coronavirus Vaccines, Moves to Right of Trump," *Washington Post*, December 17, 2022.

398   Nabin K. Shrestha et al., "Effectiveness of the Coronavirus Disease (COVID-19) Bivalent Vaccine," medRxiv preprint, December 19, 2022, https://www.medrxiv.org/content/10.1101/2022.12.17.22283625v1.full.pdf

399   Tomokazu Tamura et al., "Virological Characteristics of the SARS-CoV-2 XBB Variant Derived from Recombination of Two Omicron Subvariants," medRxiv preprint, December 19, 2022, https://www.biorxiv.org/content/10.1101/2022.12.27.521986v1

400   Zachary Stieber, "EXCLUSIVE: CDC Finds Hundreds of Safety Signals for Pfizer and Moderna COVID-19 Vaccines," *Epoch Times*, January 3, 2023, https://www.theepochtimes.com/health/exclusive-cdc-finds-hundreds-of-safety-signals-for-pfizer-and-moderna-covid-19-vaccines_4956733.html

401   Alex Berenson, "From the Twitter Files: Pfizer Board Member Scott Gottlieb Secretly Pressed Twitter to Hide Posts Challenging His Company's Massively Profitable Covid Jabs," Substack, January 9, 2023, https://alexberenson.substack.com/p/pfizer-board-member-scott-gottlieb

402   David M. Morens et al., "Rethinking Next-Generation Vaccines for Coronaviruses, Influenzaviruses, and Other Respiratory Diseases," *Cell Host & Microbe* 31, no. 1 (January 11, 2023): 146-157, https://doi.org/10.1016/chom.202211.06

Acknowledgments

Grateful acknowledgement is made to each of the following:

To the experts who generously gave of their time to make this book possible: Aditi Bhargava, Peter Breggin, Peter Doshi, David Healy, Brook Jackson, Linda Wastila, and Jenin Younes;

To Brianne and Kim, who courageously shared their stories of medical harm;

To Robert Jacobson, Ph.D., who kindly copy-edited this manuscript;

To the staff of Medstar Union Memorial Hospital, who provided me with expert, compassionate care during my hour of need;

To Theodore Houk, M.D., a man who understands the meaning of the dictum *primum non nocere*;

And to my wife and daughter, for their unwavering support.

About the Author

Patrick D Hahn is a free-lance writer and independent scholar with a long-standing interest in iatrogenic harm and the medicalization of everyday life.

His first book, *Madness and Genetic Determinism: Is Mental Illness in Our Genes?*, explores how genetic determinist views of so-called "mental illness" have obscured the well-established role of childhood sexual abuse and other adverse childhood experiences in the genesis of those conditions.

His second book, *Prescription for Sorrow: Antidepressants, Suicide, and Violence*, traces the history of how so-called "antidepressants" came on to the market and have stayed on the market, detailing how the drug companies and the mostly compliant mainstream media have exaggerated the benefits and hidden the harms caused these drugs, which include addiction, suicide, and violence.

His third book, *Obedience Pills: ADHD and the Medicalization of Childhood* discusses the harms and the lack of efficacy for the drugs commonly prescribed for the diagnostic category known as "ADHD," along with the nexus of interlocking special interests that sustains this twenty-billion-dollar-a-year industry.

Dr. Hahn is an Affiliate Professor of Biology at Loyola University Maryland.

Made in the USA
Monee, IL
30 January 2024

52657306R00197